PRAISE FOR
Being (Sick) Enough

"Through the depths of trauma, Graham emerges a radiant beacon of healing and hope for a better future. We are fortunate to bask in their brilliance!"

—JEFFREY MARSH, best-selling author of *Take Your Own Advice*

"As someone who has survived developmental trauma and understands its deep impact on the body, it's refreshing to hear such an honest voice share personal stories of their own traumatic past."

—TAMARA LEVITT, author, and head of Mindfulness at Calm

"Jessica Graham's fierce and beautiful voice pierced through these pages and straight into my heart, where it'll remain."

—JENNIFER PASTILOFF, best-selling author of *On Being Human*

"A raw and honest look at surviving trauma and navigating chronic illness and pain as a neurodivergent person while still living life to its fullest. This book avoids toxic positivity while exploring the nonlinear path of recovery, resolution, and learning to love yourself. Graham's confessional writing is grounded yet lyrical, weaving together snapshots of their lived experience in a way that entertains, inspires, and makes those of us who have ever found ourselves temporarily down for the count feel a little less alone."

—ANDREA OWEN, best-selling author of *Make Some Noise*

"A profoundly beautiful and personal work that explores the intersection of complex trauma, chronic illness, and neurodivergence. As a trauma therapist, I thought, 'Finally!' I could not help but think of all the many individuals who will likely feel validated and seen by this brave and searing account. I highly recommend this book for anyone who seeks to have a greater understanding of mental health and chronic pain."

—LAUREN MAHER, LMFT, licensed psychotherapist and author of *Mindfulness Workbook for Panic Attacks*

"Graham describes how to apply a range of mindfulness techniques—such as 'divide and conquer,' 'equanimity with pleasure and pain,' and 'connection through compassion'—to mend deep wounding from early life trauma. A rare and valuable resource!"

—SHINZEN YOUNG, meditation teacher and author of *The Science of Enlightenment*

"Graham acknowledges their limited understanding of trauma from a perspective of white privilege, recognizes the additional traumas faced by marginalized communities, and emphasizes the complexity of blame and the shared pain within their lineage—highlighting the importance of personal responsibility for healing. It's refreshing to read about sexual health from someone who has chosen to share their personal journey with such vulnerability."

—SUZANNE SINATRA, sexual health advocate and founder and CEO of Private Packs

Being (Sick) Enough

ALSO BY JESSICA GRAHAM

Good Sex: Getting Off without Checking Out

Being (Sick) Enough

THOUGHTS ON INVISIBLE ILLNESS, CHILDHOOD TRAUMA, AND LIVING WELL WHEN SURVIVING IS HARD

Jessica Graham

North Atlantic Books
Huichin, unceded Ohlone land
Berkeley, California

Published by
North Atlantic Books
Huichin, unceded Ohlone land
Berkeley, California

Cover design by Amanda Weiss
Book design by Happenstance Type-O-Rama
Author photo by Shayan Asgharnia

Printed in Canada

Being (Sick) Enough: Thoughts on Invisible Illness, Childhood Trauma, and Living Well When Surviving Is Hard is sponsored and published by North Atlantic Books, an educational nonprofit based in the unceded Ohlone land Huichin (Berkeley, CA) that collaborates with partners to develop cross-cultural perspectives; nurture holistic views of art, science, the humanities, and healing; and seed personal and global transformation by publishing work on the relationship of body, spirit, and nature.

DISCLAIMER: This book contains material that may be activating, including references to self-harm, disordered eating, addiction, sexual abuse, or trauma. The author acknowledges that certain events and conversations may have been reconstructed to the best of their ability and understanding. Names, locations, and timelines may have been altered for privacy or narrative purposes. Additionally, the perspectives presented are those of the author and may not reflect the viewpoints of others involved in the recounted events.

DISCLAIMER: The following information is intended for general information purposes only. The publisher does not advocate illegal activities but does believe in the right of individuals to have free access to information and ideas. Any application of the material set forth in the following pages is at the reader's discretion and is their sole responsibility.

MEDICAL DISCLAIMER: The following information is intended for general information purposes only. Individuals should always see their health care provider before administering any suggestions made in this book. Any application of the material set forth in the following pages is at the reader's discretion and is their sole responsibility.

North Atlantic Books's publications are distributed to the US trade and internationally by Penguin Random House Publisher Services. For further information, visit our website at www.northatlanticbooks.com.

Library of Congress Cataloging-in-Publication Data

Names: Graham, Jessica, 1980- author.
Title: Being (sick) enough : thoughts on invisible illness, childhood
  trauma, and living well when surviving is hard / Jessica Graham.
Description: Berkeley, CA : North Atlantic Books, [2024] | Includes
  bibliographical references.
Identifiers: LCCN 2024012827 (print) | LCCN 2024012828 (ebook) | ISBN
  9798889840008 (trade paperback) | ISBN 9798889840015 (ebook)
Subjects: LCSH: Graham, Jessica, 1980- | Chronically ill—United
  States—Biography. | Adult child abuse victims—United
  States—Biography. | Fibromyalgia—United States. | Post-traumatic
  stress disorder—United States.
Classification: LCC RC108 .G73 2024 (print) | LCC RC108 (ebook) | DDC
  616/.044092 [B]—dc23/eng/20240829
LC record available at https://lccn.loc.gov/2024012827
LC ebook record available at https://lccn.loc.gov/2024012828

1 2 3 4 5 6 7 8 9 MARQUIS 30 29 28 27 26 25

For the amazing humans who allow me to support them on their trauma-resolution and post-traumatic growth journeys. I am infinitely inspired by your bravery and resilience.

CONTENTS

When You Don't Think You Can Survive It

When you don't think you can't survive it
start where you are.

This is my foot on the floor.
This is my other foot tucked under my leg on the couch.
This is the sound of the heater.
This is the smell of unwashed dishes in the sink.
This is the feeling of both feet on the floor.
This is the feeling of standing up.
This is the feeling of walking across the room.
This is the sound of socked feet on hardwood.
This is what the kitchen looks like.
This is what the sink of dishes looks like.

I'm turning on the water.
I'm rinsing the crumbs and honey from this plate.
I'm opening the dishwasher.
I'm placing this plate in the dishwasher.

I'm rinsing the ring of coffee from this chipped white mug.
I'm fitting this mug into the top rack.
I'm feeling the warm water on my hands.
I'm smelling the citrus of the dish soap.

So:

I must be breathing.
I must be moving.
I must be alive.
I must be surviving.

You won't always be solely surviving. I promise you.
There are days of unfiltered joy yet to come.
There are moments when you'll say aloud, in awe and wonder,

I had no idea. I didn't realize. Thank you. Thank you.

There are new loves, and old friends, and babies to hold,
and your next favorite film to watch, and meals
that reveal once unknown layers of pleasure, and
quiet afternoons when there is nothing you have to do
except what you want to do,
and songs that you play hundreds of times a month, and a
new touch from known hands
that robs you of your breath and teaches you to breathe again.

And one day, your feet on the floor,
you'll walk to the kitchen, turn on the water,
rinse crumbs and honey from a plate, and you'll
know you survived for this simple human moment,
this miracle of being, this starting that is always
starting again.

My Parents' Hell

A little girl with brown curls, crumpled at the bottom of a long shining wooden staircase. Her mommy, beautiful and cruel at the landing above, still angry enough to fly down the stairs and deliver a final blow by way of a kick to the child's soft, round belly. The girl wears corduroy and thick cotton and still has the book she was reading in a nail-bitten hand. She doesn't know what she did or didn't do to make Mommy mad that afternoon. She floats up, up, up above the body that is curled like a snail on the floor. Another girl, younger, watching from the crack of a door, is statue-still. Mommy never hurts her, but inside she feels snail shaped anyway. Her eyes burn with all that they have seen in this pretty house, on this pretty lane. Guilt gathers in her hands, and she covers her face. The girl on the floor, now back in her body, not feeling the pain just yet, doesn't move a muscle. Silently, lips folded in, she prays for her father to come home and for her mommy to go back to the hospital.

Now: I sob as I write this opening line. I rub my tears, but they don't go away. My eyes start to sting as the sunscreen from this morning finds its way into my lower lips. I tell my tiny scruffy service dog, who is at the ready to comfort, *I'm okay, boy. I'm okay.*

A boy with hair that has been cropped short, no matter how much he begged them to let it grow, sits silently at the bright yellow kitchen table as his mother drifts further and further away into gray clouds of barbiturates and warm vodka. He has small scabs on his scalp, where the barber buzzed too close to the skin, and bruises on his arms where his mother dug in fingers to hold him still. When she places his dinner dish in front of him, the chicken is pale pink. He knows better than to name its rawness and eats the overcooked, mushy, sugary canned peas, slipping the meat into his pocket wrapped in a cloth napkin. His older brother has already cast off any role of savior and disappeared into the walls of a university 2,000 miles away. His little sister is pulled tight on Daddy's lap, his hips moving and only one hand on the wheel, in the family car that his mother never drives. They get ice cream when Daddy is done, and when he tucks her in, she can still taste the vanilla and chocolate swirl soft-serve on her tongue. When he hears her quiet tears from the next room, the boy pushes the ache of guilt down into his pocket where he keeps raw chicken and a lock of his hair, swiped from the tile floor of the barbershop.

Now: I'm no longer sobbing, but I can feel the place my pain usually starts wake up. My right shoulder blade beginning to lock and send ropes of tension down my arm. I stretch and try to relax. My dog is asleep now.

I have slices of these stories. My memory and imagination create a Rolodex of what my parents experienced at the hands of their parents. The slices I have of their parents' hells, or their parents' parents', are almost nonexistent, but there are tiny bites. My strong suspicion is that if I could take a time-bending cruise and witness the lives of my ancestors, I'd find generation after generation of trauma, and the chronic illness, mental illness, and addiction that almost invariably accompany it. Then there is the trauma of being human, regardless of how the blows are delivered. We are all, for example, traumatized by the systems that harm, such as white supremacy and the myriad evils it has bestowed upon humanity. To a certain extent, we cannot divorce ourselves entirely from some level of trauma, and the consequences of trauma, no matter how idyllic our lives have been.

These hells were all experienced inside the privilege of white bodies. As I work to resolve my own generational trauma, I aim to honor and validate my own experience while simultaneously under-standing that I can never understand what it's like to be a person living in a body that is not white. My bloodlines flow primarily from Ireland and the United Kingdom. When my ancestors emigrated to America, along with their jam-packed steamer trunks and hopes for a better life, they carried the privilege of whiteness. Over a hundred years later, that leg up has extended to me. I could go on, but the bottom line is, my pain is taken more seriously because of the color of my skin. I've received superior care because my ancestors claimed the socially constructed mantle of whiteness. Better pain management is obviously just one of the many ways my skin affords me privilege in this world. I cannot begin to know any of the hells of humans in non-white bodies; people who my maternal great-grandmother, Grammy, casually used racial slurs to describe, no matter how many times we corrected her.

Grammy came of age during the Great Depression. She got polio as a child and was partially paralyzed on one side of her body. She walked about her carpeted home in her special Grammy way, deliv-ering cheese and Lebanon bologna on white bread and butterscotch candies to me and my sisters. And yet she abused my grandmother terribly; in what ways I do not know. Grammy was an adolescent when the stock market collapsed—such formative years to experience such devastation, not to mention her disability. Her father was, in her words, a "drunken hobo" who left her mother with a slew of young children and went on to die, if the story is true, on train tracks.

I have no stories from my maternal grandfather's side. I know he stopped drinking, cold turkey, when my mother was young. I don't know how his drinking days expressed, or what traumas he endured when he was young. My grandfather loved my grandmother deeply. Once, after my grandmother surprisingly picked up a nasty drinking habit in her late sixties, he called me crying. He said he was too old for this, that it wasn't fair. When I suggested he leave, it was as if I was suggesting he remove his own heart with rusty shears. He didn't leave until the Crohn's disease he'd had since his forties made him leave, a few feet of intestines at a time.

My paternal grandmother, who I never met, died young from the long, slow death of an alcohol and drug addiction. She drank and took pills until her liver finally gave out. She let her liver rest a few times, with plans to stop the progression of cirrhosis, but ultimately oblivion was a sweeter siren than the song of life. My grandfather had another wife in Thailand. I most likely have half uncles and aunts, and maybe one day I'll get a message from 23 and Me expanding my family tree. The story goes, my grandmother drank herself to death over the heart-break of his betrayal. There have been choked and fractured whispers, from my father before he died, and then from my aunt who is now many layers deep into MAGA and, I suspect, her own alcoholism, that my grandfather sexually abused her. My paternal grandfather and aunt moved to Germany after my grandmother died, leaving my father at the young age of sixteen on his own. My uncle, my father's older brother, left home as soon as he could and has done very well for himself financially. As for money buying happiness, I can't say, I don't know him.

I remember playing with the crepey and veiny hanging skin of a very old woman's arms at a family reunion when I was five: my father's grandmother. Gran Daddy Graham was my father's grandfather, and he must have been there too. I can see his long face and round glasses in the back shelves of my memory. I don't know anything about them other than I wasn't scared of them, which says something as I was an intuitive kid. I wasn't scared of my mother's mother, or her mother, either. For me they were safe harbors, not the treacherous waters they were for their daughters. My maternal grandmother, now late in her life, has always been a support to me and is still someone with whom I feel safe and loved.

I know nothing about my paternal grandmother's side of the family, other than the fact that according to 23 and Me, she was *not* half

Cherokee as my father and 'Merica-loving aunt told me all my life. I don't need to know any details to make an educated guess that she lived through her own hell as a child. Drinking oneself to death before the age of forty tends to be preceded by a fair amount of trauma, beyond an unfaithful husband.

I know for a fact that my lineage of mothers and fathers is marred by trauma and all that comes with it, and I am unable to place the blame for the body and mind I have on any one person. I come from hurt people, and many of them have hurt people. I come from a little girl who was thrown down a flight of stairs, and a little boy who watched his mother slowly kill herself. And behind them are more hurt children who had children. While it's been important for me to temporarily assign blame and allow my anger and grief to fully arise, it's impossible to do so for long without that blame falling into a rabbit hole of the past. My pain belongs to me, to my parents, and to too many to ever name or know.

While not yet conclusive, there is growing scientific evidence that the impact of our parents' hells can be passed down through intergenerational trauma.[1] Studies suggest that children may be affected by their parents' trauma while in utero, and even before the sperm meets the egg. Furthermore, research on PTSD and epigenetics points to the possibility that trauma can affect DNA function and gene transcription for generations.[2] This potentially inherited PTSD, added to one's own lived adverse experiences, can then go on to negatively impact physical and mental health in many ways.[3] In a historical study, people who were exposed to the Dutch Hunger Winter (a period of famine in the Netherlands at the end of WW2) while in the womb were shown to be at higher risk for type 2 diabetes and schizophrenia[4] and had shorter lifespans, depending on what stage of the pregnancy their parent was in during the famine.[5] There has been ongoing study of how the children of Holocaust survivors may be genetically impacted, even though they were conceived after the war.[6] There is still much to be scientifically proven, but all signs seem to point to intergenerational trauma and its effects being very real. Personally, I don't need scientific proof to believe that chronic pain and illness erupt in the bodies of people from a family consistently eclipsed by trauma. It makes perfect sense that the traumatic events of the generational lines I come from could have something to do with my autoimmune disease, interstitial cystitis, fibromyalgia, and many of my other chronic conditions.

The pain that has held permanent residence inside my body for as long as I can remember was my unwanted, unasked-for birthright. I carried the physical and psychological traumas of my family before my face had begun to form. My amygdala, albeit primitive, already learning the dance of freeze, fight, flight, and fawn, in the rough waters of the womb. My immune system tattooed with markers as it formed. My lineage living in migraines, aching joints, burning bladder, chronic fatigue, inflamed stomach lining, ceaseless and painful muscle tension, anxiety, and depression. My body, an abstract painting or patchwork quilt of all who came before me. My addictions and disordered eating, the fine bone china and ornate silver candelabras of my inherited estates of trauma. These gifts that cannot be given back, only regifted, again and again. Regifted until someone stops the cycle.

I have hope that this cycle can end entirely, but the disease in my family tree started in the seed and has many branches. Even the young green leaves seem to be affected by the sickness of the roots. I see the discoloration in the tiniest of them, and my heart cracks, struck by the lighting of recognition, of guilt, of seeming inevitability.

And yet hope remains. I've seen how healing can happen. I do not hold this weight alone. They hold it with me, and with each generation we have learned to carry the weight with less destruction. Hope is also present in research suggesting that comprehensive trauma and attachment-based interventions, spanning individual to societal levels, can be successful in reducing the "transmission" of generational trauma.[7] I hope that one day we have billboards and public service announcements about preventing the contraction of trauma, just like we do for sexually transmitted infections and the flu.

Resolving my personal trauma, along with the trauma of those who came before me, has been my life's work. It has been a literal bloody mess at times. It has been heartbreaking, and despair ridden. But this work has also been full of beauty, awakening, and love. The progress I've made (and seen many of my family members make) so far is my greatest accomplishment and has led to a profound sense of purpose and meaning, through service to others on this healing path.

Sometimes healing is simply the acceptance of what is and the welcoming of what comes next. Sometimes it's more tangible, more concrete. Sometimes healing finds its ways into the deepest layers of earth. Sometimes I swear I can feel the hands of a little girl with brown curls and a boy with a scabbed scalp in mine. I hold on tight. We run and run. We don't look back. We laugh like real children, because we are.

Being Santa's Child-Parent

I was six when I found out there was no Santa Claus and learned that I was my father's surrogate parent.

We slept in a *family bed,* which meant two queen-size mattresses on the floor. That nest of sheets and blankets provided a sleeping place for me, my mother, my dad, my four-year-old sister, and my little baby sister, just a few months old.

It was Christmas Eve, and I was six, so obviously I couldn't sleep. We had left out chips and salsa for the fat jolly white man. I imagine it would be hard to avoid leaving a splattering of red tomato on that giant mass of silvery white facial hair. Santa eating salsa might look like a well-fed vampire—with a penchant for gift wrapping and reindeer. Maybe that's why the traditional snack is milk and cookies, rather than the spicy Pace Picante that my parents suggested that night.

I was listening for any sound of hooves on the roof, or perhaps a friendly, hushed *Ho, ho, ho*. We didn't have a fireplace, so I'm not sure why Santa would have landed on our roof. But that didn't concern me. What concerned me was the joyful energy running through my little body, squeezed between my mother and my dad in the family bed. I was buzzing with the hope that there was something to look forward to the next morning. And it wouldn't be on my parents' dime. Santa was footing this bill.

I knew that money was tight because I had recently witnessed my dad swallowing his pride, not for the first time, to ask his rich brother for a loan. My dad was working toward membership in Local 13, a union of boilermakers who spent their days in oil refineries. He still had a ways to go before decent pay and a spot on the top of the list, so he was dependent on short-term odd jobs. One time our next-door neighbor, who (allegedly) had a very lucrative business bringing cocaine into the country and dispensing it, gave my dad $600 to paint his bathroom. That was a lot of money in the early '80s, and my dad told me that the bathroom wasn't even in need of fresh paint. Our neighbor, who had snarly guard dogs and beautiful peacocks behind the massive walls around his house, knew we were struggling and just wanted to put some money in my dad's pocket. My mother took care of me and my sisters while also collecting odd jobs herself, mostly domestic labor such as cleaning house and childcare.

Compared to us, and to most people honestly, my uncle was loaded. We heard about his tennis courts, his jet, his thriving spinal surgery practice. We heard about how, at age eighteen, he left my dad and his younger sister, after their mother had died of cirrhosis, never to return. We heard about how square he was. No following Led Zeppelin around the country. No peyote buttons with a shaman in New Mexico. He wore a suit and tie to go to dinner on a Tuesday night. He belonged to several country clubs. He *golfed*. And he left a big-brother size hole in my dad's heart when he cut and ran, looking for a better life than what his family of origin could offer.

I don't remember when I first saw my dad cry about the loss of his brother. My dad's tears were commonplace from the beginning of my life. He cried to me when I was six and my mother was moving out, with my sisters and me in tow. He cried to me when I was eleven and he called to let me know he would miss my twelfth birthday because he'd be in rehab. He cried to me when I was thirteen and he told me he had gotten another DUI while passed out in his car on the side of the road. He cried to me when I was fourteen and he was headed to jail for ten days. He cried when I was sixteen and he begged me to come home after we'd had a big fight and I disappeared for days. Later he cried to me when he got his cancer diagnosis, when he got ninety days sober and drank again, when he was home alone, starving and struggling with his feeding tube, surrounded by years of stacked newspapers, active rodent nests, and bagless trash cans filled with soiled adult diapers and beer cans. His suffering was a tsunami. He nearly drowned me in tears and pleas for advice.

If, instead of his child, he had cried to a professional, or even just a caring adult, things may have been very different. He might have gotten sober for good. He might have turned all his potential into a beautiful life, maybe not as luxurious a life as his brother's, but comfortable and safe. I might not have learned that money is something that other people have. I might have learned that there was enough for us too.

Growing up below the poverty line for periods of time made me see people like my uncle (and our drug-peddling neighbor) like mythical creatures, or royal beings who lived in a stone and steel castle, behind moats and gates and guards. People with money were either yuppies (one of the worst insults my dad could sling, a close second to *Republican*) or they were rich like my uncle.

Yuppies could be seen in the wild, but rich people were hard to come by. My parents bought a house in an area that was on the verge of gentrification (aka a bunch of white people were about to converge). There was a diverse socioeconomic landscape on our street. Some neighbors were in a similar position to our family, some were more financially secure, and some were yuppies who had granite countertops in their kitchens. They had human-made ponds in their backyards, home to turtles, frogs, and maybe even giant colorful koi fish. Some of them weren't all that bad for yuppies, my dad said. They enjoyed the Rolling Stones and Tabasco sauce on their eggs (hollandaise was sacrilege). They invited our scrappy feral family, clothed in Goodwill and smelling of Ivory soap, dust, and possibly cannabis, to their cookouts and crab bakes, and even to the annual egg hunts where the women wore big fancy Easter hats. One year, my dad put us all in hard hats borrowed from a stint at the oil refinery. He took photos of me and my sisters for as long as he was physically able, and there exists somewhere a picture of us in our Easter hard hats, ready to collect plastic eggs full of candy.

I once found the *golden egg* at one of those hunts. The golden egg awarded the winner a trip to the workshop of the town tie-dyer, to choose any t-shirt there. The town tie-dyer was not a yuppie. She was a dyed-in-the-wool hippie. But she also had a pool. A pool should have pushed her into yuppie territory, but her long undyed hair, bangles on her wrists, sleepy style of speaking, and the multicolored clothing that she sold out of her home studio and at music festivals and art shows allowed her to retain the hippie title with my dad, and therefore with me.

Looking through the racks of rainbowed cotton made me forget about money, or lack thereof. I could choose anything from the tie-dye workshop that I wanted—only people with money got to do that. One of these amazing shirts would be mine.

Along with the excitement, I was feeling a little guilty. *I* hadn't actually found the golden egg. My dad had stealthily pointed it out to me. He had a true St. Nick twinkle in his eyes, as his finger directed me to the jumbo plastic egg, painted gold, nestled under the rhododendron. Was it just what some parents do? Helping their kids succeed at life, even if a little cheating is involved? Or was it the kid inside my dad who never really got to be a kid who pointed out the golden egg? His early life was no holiday. He didn't have the luxury of much childlike fun. When the excitement of catching sight of the golden egg rushed through my body, did my dad feel it in the empty places where his childhood would have been? My good feelings becoming an imagined memory of his?

My dad wanted me to feel good. When I felt good, he felt good. I believe that he rejoiced when I hit the magic age of fourteen and could be his late-night companion. That must have been the age he was when he started drinking, smoking, and doing drugs; that's how old I was when he was supplying me with alcohol, buying me cigarettes, and hosting me and my friends at his efficiency apartment for all-nighters. That's what made me feel good, what made him feel good. There is a photo that he took of me and a friend one afternoon, passed out head to feet on the couch. We are in our clothes from the night before, our baby faces sweaty and flushed, surrounded by empty bottles of beer and wine coolers. He had been up with us all night, playing classic rock records and telling stories of his youth. Borrowing from our youth. Drinking in my vibrance, while I drank the drinks he poured, until my vibrance dimmed. When I woke that day, he likely suggested "hair of the dog" to cure my hangover, as he often did and which inevitably led to a repeat of the night before.

My dad had lost all his friends due to his alcoholism. I offered him another chance at belonging. Until I was eighteen, he was a fixture in my circle of friends. Every so often he would get so embarrassingly drunk that I'd have to lock him out of the room we were in. But usually he danced and sang with us in the living room, which was his bedroom, in the apartment we rented together. He cooked us Spam and beans at 3 a.m. when we got the munchies. He got into political and philosophical conversations with us, over shared cases of Budweiser and packs of Marlboro Reds. It was incredibly hard for him when I started wanting a social life of my own. Surprisingly, he was mostly supportive when I quit drinking. He was proud of my sobriety. Perhaps that too was something he could imagine as his. His was a life lived vicariously.

He loved inhabiting my life and had difficulty seeing me as separate from him. Even my hair was somehow his. This started as early as I can remember. My mother once had my bangs cut and he was furious. I had his thick hair; how dare she chop it off into such a silly style. Later when I wanted to get under his skin I would threaten to get my hair thinned out and he would read me the riot act. When I was seventeen and shaved my head, I recall him actually crying a bit. He handled my body as if it belonged to him. Inappropriately tender cuddles that I had to fight my way out of. Kisses on the lips when I said no. Relentless tickle attacks that left me no choice but to punch and kick until he yelped in pain and let me go.

My romantic life served as a surrogate for him too, as he pretty much stopped dating before I was a teenager. He had no qualms with asking me (or the people I dated) about my sex life or telling me explicit details about his past exploits. He tended to form inappropriately strong attachments to the people I dated, especially a few of the men. He once took a multiweek road trip with two of the men I had dated, both under twenty-one. When I unexpectedly broke up with one of them, my dad was irrationally angry. He told me I had no class and that he never thought I could be that kind of person. It took my dad longer to forgive me than it did my ex-boyfriend. His high school girlfriend had unceremoniously broken up with him too. He wanted me to offer an alternative version of his first love, rather than residing in the reality where his heart was still broken decades later. My dad carried the pain of that breakup, and every one after it, his entire life. Just as he carried the pain of his childhood trauma in his body.

My dad had chronic pain just like me. Bone of my bone. Flesh of my flesh. He passed it to me in a billion little torches. When you add a flame to a flame, you don't get two flames, you get a bigger flame. One plus one is one. The burning and aching bonfire that moved through my dad's muscles and joints and stomach now move through mine. I spent my childhood trying to birth him into parenthood. Trying to breathe him into being a dad, and instead breathed him into my being. His pain, my pain.

Maybe his pointing out that golden egg hidden among the foliage all those Easters ago was just a parent eager to see their child's delighted smile. Maybe it was the beginnings of what would later be his pointing out the last beer, hidden behind a brown bag of leftovers in the back of the fridge, delighting in letting me have it. Whatever the reason, my dad's discovery of that egg that led to my all-time favorite t-shirt. It had dark curved lines running right along where my ribs would be. A skeleton tie-dye. I loved it until I lost it. It flew off the roof of the car, inside my rainbow suitcase, that had been forgotten when the trunk was packed after a camping trip with my family and a man and his sons we had befriended. My dad went back and looked on the highway later that week but only found the suitcase, empty and torn. When you don't have much, one lost tie-dyed shirt, even one that you didn't win fair and square, is worth grieving.

No matter how much you have, a lost brother is also worth grieving. I imagine what my dad might have thought to himself as a small boy when his big brother left, no one else to say it to:

Does he remember the train set that we spent hours constructing and breaking down and reconstructing? Does he remember that my favorite train was the blue caboose and his was the car marked "oranges"? Did he see my face on the other side of the slammed screen door, willing him to stay?

My dad longed for his big brother to be part of his life. He longed for his dead mother, his distant father, and his sister who he eventually became estranged from due to alcoholism and vast political divides. His longing was not relieved. There was no path back to a family that never really existed. Sometimes I would come home, and the lights would be low, my dad sitting in the middle of the room, cigarette smoke dancing around him, drunken tears soaking his face, listening to "Mother," John Lennon's heart-wrenching song about being abandoned by his parents, on repeat. So lost in his own longing and sorrow, he couldn't see that history was repeating in my practically parentless life. I played out the very same scene, with the very same soundtrack, a few times myself.

My dad showed parental love through money—if he couldn't buy love, he could at least use cash as a stand-in. When my dad had money in the bank, he loved spending it on me and my sisters. He took us on annual road trips to Florida, giving us coffee cans full of a year's worth of pocket change to pack into paper rolls and cash in for a stack of bills to spend along the way. I got a crisp Benjamin for my twelfth birthday. I remember being wide eyed and positively thrilled. He was always ready to pay for a meal or a movie. I got to ride all the rides when the fair came to town. After I moved to Los Angeles, my dad showed his love by sending me drugstore greeting cards with a twenty-dollar bill tucked in with a note to "buy an avocado sandwich." He also paid for my car insurance for a few years and sent me enough money to buy twenty-five avocado sandwiches when I ran into a lean period.

Just a few months before he died, I was visiting him at the hospital when he asked me to help him and his IV take a walk to the lobby. When we arrived, after a slow journey down halls and elevators, he beelined for the ATM. He took out a wad of cash and, stuffing it in my hands, asked in a surgery-ravaged croak of a voice, *Is that enough?* I asked, *For what, Dad?* He replied, *I just want to make sure you are okay for money while you are here.* I tried to give it back, but he refused. This was how he could show me love, so I pocketed the money, and we started the long trip back to his hospital room.

My golfing, spine-slicing, chiropractor-hating uncle, who I met once at two months and once a few days before my father died, didn't realize that my dad asking for another loan was my dad asking for his love. Or maybe he did, in some back corner of his mind, in some place behind all the anger and resolve. Either way, when my dad slammed down the orangey-red rotary phone that Christmas, I knew that his brother wasn't going to pay out.

Years later, my uncle financially supported me while I cared for my dying dad. He made it possible for me to wash my dad's body the day before he died, to breathe with him for his last night of breath, to hold my sister's hands as we sat stunned and sleep deprived the next day. I don't care if it was guilt money or not, I was grateful. I think my dad was too, and maybe it made up for that day his brother said *no*, through the rotary phone, to being Santa Claus with a sack full of money ready to dole out loans with no hope of repayment.

My dad made a Santa of my mother after she left, unable to live with his drinking and in love with the man who had joined us on the family camping trip when I lost my tie-dye t-shirt. She was his Santa every time he missed another child support payment. When she was forced to sell their house, rather than let the investment mature, because he swore to her that he would let it go to ruin unless she came back. When she invited him to spend his last months in her home, where she lived with the man from the camping trip.

He made a Santa of me too. When I was fourteen and he sold all my CDs to pay his bills and keep himself drunk. When I was fifteen and paying rent in our basement apartment. When I paid a friend to check on him and take him food, because I had moved to Los Angeles and he told me he wasn't eating and that he had passed out in a snowbank one night the week before and woke up freezing, bleeding, and missing the cash from his wallet. When I put the beer he begged for in his feeding tube, because he could no longer swallow even liquid. I was his Santa, his child-parent, when I tried to cheer him up with hugs and kisses on the lips the day his brother refused to bail him out yet again, and I saw his heart break as the phone smashed into the receiver.

My dad had a way of getting more drunk than usual on holidays. He was hard to wake up. On Christmas Eve 1985, my mother gave up on my dad and left him in bed. He wasn't going to wake up, she'd have to wrap the presents in the last few weeks of the funny pages on her own. There would only be her gray fingerprints of last week's newspaper on the scotch tape.

After my mother moved us out, we went for overnights with my dad. Once the youngest of us was there on her own. A toddler, she could walk and talk, but she couldn't wake up dad. At only two or three, my baby sister told our mother that she didn't want to sleep over anymore after that. Not me, I fought tooth and nail to watch my dad get drunk and fall asleep on the floor every weekend. I'd probably do the same today, given the option. It'd be nice to see him again, even unconscious.

I was my dad's biggest fan. He was smart, handsome, and hilarious. He could name the Academy Award–winning film of almost every year, and many of the best performer and director recipients too. He loved films and music and could converse on most genres and styles. He understood and could explain complex sociopolitical issues. He loved science of all kinds. He could dance and wasn't embarrassed to do so, even when he wasn't drunk. He had a profound connection to nature and made it a priority to spend time exploring up until he got too sick to travel. He was fiercely loyal to the people he loved. Children adored him and he would keep playing freeze tag or touch football long after the other adults tired. He was a good writer (I begged him to write more of his stories before he died, but he only filled a few pages of the notebook I bought him). He started painting desert landscapes on cardboard canvases cut from cases of beer in the last few years of his life. He had the heart of an artist and the mind of a philosopher.

My dad had potential. That potential was a siren for me and kept me in the role of his cheerleader, Santa Claus, and stand-in parent until he died. If I loved him hard enough, he would wake from the spell of trauma and addiction and become the dad he was always meant to be, but not just that. He would become the person he was meant to be, all that potential made manifest. As an adult, all good sense told me that I didn't hold this power or this responsibility, but that didn't change my mission to love him until he could love himself. I claimed the emotional burden of his unresolved trauma. I chose him over me, as he chose death over me. With each drink, cigarette, missed meal, and denial of basic human needs, he gave up.

I didn't give up. I was carrying my dad's heart in my heart, his body was my body, and I didn't give up on him until the hospital sent him home for the last time. Even then, I held his bones wrapped in gray skin close to me in his hospice bed. I willed myself to merge with him, letting go of the edges and boundaries. A last-ditch effort to bring him to life through me. Bone of my bones. Flesh of my flesh.

I thought I couldn't survive my dad's death. I didn't know how to exist without him in the world. The boundary between him and me was flimsy and porous at best. Our connection seemed written in the stars. How was I expected to keep on breathing if he stopped? It was my job to take care of him, to entertain him, to be his companion and confidant. What purpose would I have if he were gone?

As a young adult I tried to quit that job, and I erected rigid boundaries between me and my dad. I had no patience for his drunkenness or tears. I refused to give him advice or let him be part of my social sphere. I stopped going on vacations to Florida with him, no longer tolerating the long drives down I-95 and sharing rooms with him in cheap motels. I pretended not to notice the magical synchronicities that occurred between us. I was mean to him in ways that still make me flinch with guilt. I pushed him away at every chance, and it devastated him. I didn't know how else to breathe my own breath, to live my own life.

Then one afternoon he called me, drunk and scream-crying that he had cancer. I screamed back, wild rage covering my despair. That rage didn't keep him from dying, though I tried it again and again. I tried so many things. His cancer diagnosis put me back to work on the job I had tried to quit. If I could say the right thing, in the right way, maybe I could save him. Over the four years that his alcoholism partnered with cancer, I went from bossing him, to begging him, to limiting my time with him to half-hour visits because any more would lead to me yelling at him and then feeling guilty and ashamed. Finally, I tried to quit the job again. I barely spoke to him for months. It felt like cutting off a limb, but I was determined to hold firm. I told myself, and others, that I had said my last goodbye.

But the news from my sisters back East kept getting worse and the doctors, set on curing death, cut his voice from his throat. He was going to die. It was clear. I needed to let down the boundaries one last time. I had quit drinking and started meditating. I had new tools and skills to bring with me for this actual last goodbye. I also knew I couldn't save him, so my only job now was to love him. I let myself fall into him. His body, my body. A parent and their dying child. Only love and acceptance remained.

I knew I couldn't save him in those final months, but on that long-ago Christmas Eve I was certain I could bring him back to the world of the living, and whatever my mother needed him for—I could make him a parent.

That night, without speaking a syllable, I scooted a foot or so away from my dad, pulled my knee up to my belly, and kicked. Hard. Right in his upper thigh. I don't know why violence seemed to be the answer in that moment, but it worked. My dad woke up, grumbling, suddenly remembering what day it was, noticing that his was the only adult body in the bed. Unsure of why his leg was screaming at him, he got off the mattress and found his way along the narrow hall, and down the narrow staircase, his narrow frame shrugging off the sleep and the pain. Relieved, I went back to listening for the sound of sleigh bells.

I was relieved when my dad died. I wish he were still here and I'm glad he isn't. I watched him suffer for so long, helpless to deliver him from his pain, and yet confident that it was my sacred duty. I had given so much of my life to him, but he was like a hungry ghost. No matter how much of myself I fed him, it fell right through. I could never fill the brother-mother-father-sister-lover shaped void that made a weeping phantom of him. There are consequences of sacrificing your-self that way. There is a cost to lending your youth out to an adult who never got to be a child. Tolls must be paid to cross the River Styx when you go looking for lost souls. I lost a lot trying to find my dad. It wasn't my fault, and it wasn't his. It was a loss passed down from one parent-less child to the next.

One of the greatest losses in becoming a surrogate parent to my dad has been never getting to become a parent to a child of my own. I'm childless not by choice. I've had to trudge through the hall of mir-rors, my parents reflected in every relationship, until I cried out loud enough to shatter them all. I emerged from the shards as a true parent to myself, and to the child I never got to be. The reparenting process has proven to be a full-time job. So, while I have a niece and nephews who I adore and take endless pictures of (I took the very first photo of one, just his tiny wet head peeking out of the birth canal), I don't have a little one of my own to kick me awake, high on the thigh. No bruises from playing tickle monster in the backyard. No toes stubbed from running down streets after skinny legs and wild hair. A good kind of pain. The hazards of loving humans who don't yet know how to con-trol their bodies into behaving.

After my uncontrolled little foot kicked him awake, I listened to my dad make his way down the stairs, realizing that something was not quite right. Didn't we all have to be sleeping for Santa to bring our gifts? I strained my ears to listen to what would happen next, already bracing for my childlike faith to be broken, as it would be again and again.

The crunching of tortilla chips drifted through the floorboards like morse code. Decoded.

Floating in the Swamp of Sadness

Sweet sixteen. I sat on the linoleum tile floor of the studio apartment I shared with my dad when he was in town, back against the wall, curlicue phone cord twisted in the four fingers of my left hand, talking to the suicide prevention hotline. The man on the other end sounded like he was tall and hunched with his hair thinning at the temples. I couldn't tell if he was kind, or if it was exhaustion making his voice sound so heavy and slow. It was after midnight, not actually my birthday anymore. How long had he been answering calls like mine that night? I called to say I couldn't try anymore. I didn't care anymore.

I was alone, and not drunk enough, with a purple bruise blooming in my heart because one of my best friends was with the twenty-two-year-old man who I had been obsessed with for several years. He was a punk-rock alcoholic junkie (today, clean and sober), and he was not mine. He belonged to all of us castaway kids. We took turns playing the role of his salvation, dodging his sarcasm, kissing his pierced lips and skin covered with hand-drawn tattoos, and drinking his Wild Irish Rose with ice from a plastic thermos covered with band stickers. He never did more than fuck me with his mouth and fingers, and he wouldn't let me try heroin, no matter how convincing I was at being a grown-up. I once begged him to fuck me with his cock, rubbing up against him as we lay on a twin mattress on his bedroom floor in his parents' house. He refused, saying as much as he wanted to be inside me, he'd shared needles and wouldn't risk my health. Later that night he asked me to close my eyes while he shot up. Once when he was trying to get clean, he asked me to hide all the spoons in a Denny's booth where we were drinking hours-old coffee and chain-smoking cigarettes.

When I turned sixteen, my father, who'd done heroin a few times as a teen but liked beer more, was in Harrisburg or Pittsburgh or some other -berg. He was trying to get his driver's license back after three DUIs, ten days in jail, and over four years hiding his bike in the bushes by freeway exits where work buddies would pick him up and drive him to the oil refineries he worked in. When he was gone, I got the full mattress on the floor to myself and I spent less time in my room, which was the bathroom, where I kept bottles of liquor and clothing in the linen cabinet and sometimes put a cot in the bathtub. Sometimes I had sex on the shaggy never-laundered bathmat. Once a few friends and I sliced our thumbs open and became blood brothers, red drippings on black and white tiles. We laughed and laughed, drunk, with layers of toilet paper wrapped around our fresh wounds. When my dad was home, the bathroom gave me a place to sleep without the scent of his rotten teeth and the sadness in his eyes when I refused to cuddle.

The night of my sixteenth birthday I would have been happy to sleep with him under the polyester sheets and the purple, pink, and tan afghan handmade by a family member whose name I don't remember. I would have welcomed his bad advice and too long hugs. We would have drunk his cans of beer and smoked cigarettes and tried to keep our always loud voices quiet so that the neighbor on the other side of the shockingly thin wall wouldn't bang and shout and call the cops. My dad would have given me some cash or a classic rock CD wrapped in newspaper as a present. We wouldn't have had singing or candles, but maybe some Tastykakes and Wawa hoagies set out on ice chests and cardboard boxes. We'd sit on an outdoor folding chair and single wooden chair that sat tableless in the kitchenette where we never cooked, unless the meal came from a can.

I was not happy on my sixteenth birthday, and I'm not happy today. But that's what my mind is telling me, so it's probably not true. It's raining, which adds to the melancholy and supports my mind's opinion on how I am feeling, but still, I'm not sure I believe it. My sweet animal brain has always been fuzzy and wired for sinking into a swamp of sadness. Even then, when I celebrated my sweet sixteen, I was trying to smooth it out and rewire the neural pathways that led me again and again to despair, though I didn't fully understand that's what I was doing. I was just trying to feel better when I called the suicide hotline. It was the same thing I did as a six-year-old when I would call the Storytime hotline from our orange rotary phone, so the recorded voice of an adult could offer me comfort in the form of make-believe tales that were updated every week. On weeks when my homelife was particularly bad, I would call repeatedly, listening to the same story again and again. In both the suicide hotline and the Storytime hotline I was looking for a friend to call me out of the murky depths, like Atreyu called to rescue his loyal and loving horse Artax in *The NeverEnding Story*. "You have to try," the friend would say. "You have to care."

I *was* trying and I *did* care, and that remains the same today, on another birthday. This depression that comes upon me isn't unreasonable. It will listen to my pleas and recede if I am willing to make the effort. The practice of meditation has shown me that most of my suffering is optional and stems from the stories my mind tells me. On days like today all it takes is the willingness to stop thinking shitty thoughts to be released from it. Since gaining this insight, I've always, eventually, been willing to make the effort. Today that effort is ordering groceries, putting meat and vegetables into the crock pot, letting a friend drop off cookies even though I don't want to see anything with a face other than my dog, doing some YouTube yoga and a short meditation, reading the flood of social media birthday wishes (didn't have that when I turned sixteen), crying but not to the point of a shot nervous system, cuddling the cute-faced dog, cleaning my apartment that I don't share with anyone, counting my liters of water so that my pee runs clear not dark yellow, possibly a micro-microdose of depression-busting magic mushrooms, and remembering again and again that my mind is a liar.

My mind has historically had a knack for something called automatic negative thought. Examples of this kind of thought include all-or-nothing thinking (*I'll never be happy. I'm always miserable. I should just give up*), overgeneralizing based on a single negative experience (*That one Tinder date ghosting me is proof that I'm unattractive and unlovable*), mental filtering and disqualifying the positive by fixating on the one thing that went wrong, or discounting anything positive from an experience, jumping to painful conclusions through distorted assumptions of what the future holds, catastrophizing, making your feelings facts (*I feel like I'm not smart enough, so everyone must think I am a dummy*), and rushing to blame yourself or others for circumstances without considering all sides of the situation with mindful discernment. I don't know about you, but I'd wager a bet that 99.9 percent of such thought is pure bullshit. Hence, the need to remember that if my mind were Pinocchio, its nose would be a mile long. And wouldn't you know, childhood trauma increases the likelihood of automatic negative thoughts.[1]

The imprints of childhood trauma and masking undiagnosed autism and ADHD made my mind less than trustworthy. When everything feels like an emergency to the nervous system due to a chronic state of fight, flight, freeze, or fawn, the mind will come up with stories to make sense of what's happening in the body. When your early years are a messy layer cake of disappointment, your mind will prompt you to expect disappointment at every turn. When you've been told from a young age that you are too sensitive to stimuli, that you fidget too much, that you talk too loud or fast, that you are too messy, that you are too easily upset by a change in routine, that you are too blunt, and that you are just too weird, your mind will learn to say all those things, and worse, about you too. Your mind will lie.

After years of observing the activity of my mind through meditation, resolving big chunks of my childhood trauma, and recognizing that my neurodivergence is not a failing or even a problem, I experience almost no negative self-talk. When I have a conscious judgmental thought about myself or someone else, it's glaringly obvious, like it's coming from a megaphone. Even when it flares up and starts lying, on days like today, it's not a harsh bully. I am kind to myself now, more kind than I was when I was sixteen. But I'm also tired. I've seen my heart and mind heal and recover in countless ways. I've experienced changes at the level of the nervous system that feel miraculous. For the most part I have a beautiful and privileged life, but it's been a lot of work and the work continues. There is a young part of me that has been trying so hard for so long, and now and then they just don't wanna. Today I found myself making my bed—fresh sheets tend to help with the sinking feeling—and saying aloud, *How many times am I going to have to make a bed until this is over?* This is the kind of lie my mind tends to tell me these days. It says that life is meaningless, and that annihilation seems like a better option than this merry-go-round of the human condition. Sometimes the confluence of depression, chronic pain, and complex PTSD symptoms, plus living in a world built for a neurotypical brain, feels like burnout. It makes me feel like an office worker who hides in the bathroom at lunch eating a tuna salad sandwich and just trying to find the energy to go back out and smile at Glen in marketing on the way to their cubicle.

The only time I ever worked in an office was for a few months as the volunteer coordinator at a hospice. I'm not sure if the director knew I had never even graduated high school when she slid the hourly rate across the table on a small square of white paper and apologized for how low it was—though it wasn't low for me. I didn't last long at that job because I wanted to be at the bedside of dying people, not training others to be there. I feel comfortable and in my element in the presence of people who have already made their last bed. Aside from that, I was and remain to be far too feral for office life. I imagine my burnout is akin to what it must feel like to work day after day in an enclosed office environment, no matter how much the CEO purports to care and how many "avoiding burnout" seminars have been scheduled. It's the feeling that you will have to just keep doing this until you, hopefully, retire. This sense that no matter what you do, you'll find yourself back here in this building with gray carpet and beige walls; or back in this state of mind that wraps me in wet wool and whispers that I am trapped and alone and always will be. Those automatic negative thoughts sure are pesky fuckers, and it's no surprise that they have been shown to cause depression and anxiety.[2]

I've been working to create a new normal since before I knew that my normal was not good for living things. I go many months, even years, without the swamp of sadness pulling me to the shower floor, tears mixing with soap. I once had a baseline of mostly unconditional discontent that was littered with manic moments of cotton-candy-high happiness, laser-pointed hyperfixation, and muddy swamp-bottom misery. That is not how I live today.

I now know that I am not trapped or alone. I wouldn't say that all my days are filled with unending joy, but I have established a baseline of unconditional peace and happiness that maintains its level and continues to rise. This happy and peaceful state that is independent of conditions has been cultivated over years of meditation practice and periods of awakening. When thoughts are seen to be nothing more than impermanent phenomena, no matter how nasty they are, they can't fuck with that state of being. There is also great happiness and peace to be found when the spell of separation is broken. Knowing through and through that I am connected to everything, everywhere, for all time, in all space, delivers great freedom from the bondage of a trapped and lonely self. For me that interconnection and freedom has led to an understanding that everything is deeply, unconditionally okay, even when life feels like a meaningless fight to the death. The conditions of my day-to-day life or of the troubled world at large have ceased to be able to shake that growing foundation of peace and happiness. This has become my new normal. But wanting to stay alive still feels like work sometimes.

I am and have always been like a water-starved plant reaching for the light in a basement apartment. I keep reaching, yet still I can wilt. Haven't all of us who have listened to friendly strangers' rehearsed voices telling us to *try*, to *care,* felt like that plant sometimes? Perhaps it's all the reaching for the sun that winds me, delivers days like today, when it just seems too far to stretch. Through this lens, depression is like the pain of committing to being alive. When I make my calls to the void, which have led to calls to a hotline more than once, I am not wanting to die. Yes, at times that seemed like an excellent option, but even then I didn't want to stop living. I wanted to start living anew.

Once, when the swamp had me and was not letting up going on a year, I started googling depression and suicidal ideation. Much like when I turned sixteen, I was looking for a friend who could help me try, help me care. I found a TED talk by someone I can't remember, but I recall the speaker asked an important question: *Do you want to die, or do you just want to feel differently than you do?* It's so simple, and as someone who was already making a living helping other people want to live, it was humbling, how much it helped. I did want to feel differently. I *do* want to feel differently. This desire to feel differently can be held inside unconditional peace and happiness. It's not either-or.

Acceptance is the holy grail when it comes to allowing these seemingly opposite experiences to coexist. I need to accept that I sometimes want to feel differently than I do. It's that desire that can bring me back from the brink. That holy and human desire for contentment with oneself. The desire to sit back into and enjoy peace and happiness, knowing that all is well. The desire to *not* have to try so hard and to care easily. The desire to fast-forward to the end of the movie when Artax, who had previously succumbed to the swamp, is wished back to life and Fantasia is saved from the all-consuming nothing. This is a pure and beautiful desire, and for me, it's what these days of darker shades of gray and wet wool originate from.

When I connect with this true wanting and allow it to express fully, the swamp dries, and I can climb out and brush the cracked mud off my body with little effort. It used to take what felt like a never-ending amount of time to find my way to this connection, expression, and shift of emotional landscape. I believed everything my mind told me back then. On that sweet sixteen birthday, my mind told me that I was alone and always would be. It said I would lose what I had and never get what I wanted. My mind wove a story of a nefarious nothing that grew bigger and bigger until there was only emptiness. But somehow at the same time, I knew that there was relief, and even miraculous change, available to me.

If I think too much about it, I question the meaning of this life I've lived and why it's needed to so often be infused with sadness. This string of birthdays, some lonely and tearful, some surrounded by loved ones and smiling until it hurts, some completely forgettable. The day that marks another year of trying and caring and following the basic desire to keep living, and I'm left wondering when this plant of my life will finally be moved to a spot with just the right amount of direct sunlight.

But thanks to meditation, I don't tend to think too much about anything for very long, and that line of existential questioning sputters out before it can really take hold, and before I know it, I feel different.

Today my heart feels heavy, soft, and slow. I'm listening to it like it's a kind and tired stranger on the telephone, or favorite childhood story. The rain stopped and there is a new moon. I dipped into my stash of psilocybin, and the wet wool has been hung outside to drip-dry. I may be able to fold it up and put it in the cedar chest for a little while.

I am trying. I do care.

A Place Where Bad Things Happen

When I was fifteen, and between exiles from my mother's home, I went to public school. *Public school* was a dirty phrase in my mother's home. A place where bad things happened.

Up until then, my entire formal education had been a two-and-a-half-year, life-saving stint at a hippie school in the woods, beginning when I was nine. We sang Beatles songs in a white dome. We climbed trees and learned about Greek mythology and racism and made thick clumpy candles by dipping a long wick in tin cans of wax and then water and then wax. I fell in love with several boys, at least two girls, and one substitute teacher who was dating an artist with long braids, who had been my neighbor before my mother left my dad and we moved into a tiny basement apartment with baby roaches who became my friends. While attending this school I was frightened every time I learned something new—I felt my options were perfection or possible death, but I didn't die, and the learning was a remedy that had been withheld, and it held me until I bloomed fresh and bright.

At the end of that time of magic and morning circles and the smell of warm brown bread smeared with butter from patchy yellowed blocks, I begged (maybe on my knees?) to go on to middle school, to public school, with the other twelve-year-olds. I had also begged at four, and five, and six, and seven. By eight I stopped asking, squeezing the curiosity and wonder into a migraine-shaped box, but the next year my dream was miraculously, albeit briefly, realized when I got to attend the hippie school in the woods. I cried into thin scratchy tissues on my last day as a student there.

My rich uncle whom I'd never met offered to fund my father's fight to force my mother to allow me the privilege of continued education. But my mother's eyes could kill. My mother's hands could leave red welts on white skin and a dizzy head from meeting walls. My mother's way of erasing me erased me.

Brushing off my knees, wiping my desire down, I decided that my father's disappointment, my disappointment, was the better option compared to my mother's violent wrath and silent rage. Middle school wouldn't wait, but I would. I bloomed into someone who did things that felt safest to do; I crystallized and froze before I bled, before I knew what I was giving up when I left learning.

I waited. I was kicked out of the house at fourteen, too much sex with grown men and wine coolers and vodka in a water jug in my closet and LSD and harder things and my harder skin; I had learned to hit back with blood in my teeth after leaving red mouth-shaped marks on the white of my mother's skin.

I was a bad happening and I had no place.

After some time, she begged me (maybe on her knees?) to come back. I did, of course I did, I still wished I was a kid. My mother did not argue when I enrolled myself in public school. Maybe it was all the months she knew I'd spent fending for myself. Or that withholding love no longer had the power to hold me. Maybe it was the fact that I had proven myself a fighter, with teeth.

Sometimes when I missed the bus, I stood at the top of our driveway and stuck out a thumb. Once an old lady in a very clean car picked me up and scolded me, telling me I was a good girl and to stay in school. Once a white van with no windows and two white men with wet red mouths inside stopped, but I didn't get in. I'd been to a few rodeos by then. I knew where bad things happened.

I lasted three months in high school. I could not acclimate. I wasn't a kid. I wasn't an adult. I was feral and wise. I was jaded and limitless. I couldn't find my place, though looking back I never ate a lunch alone, I was cast in the school play, and I met the love of my life in the front row of honors English. For me it was a place where things happened: not too bad, just too late.

On my last day, the science teacher accused me of skipping class, when in fact I had been in a traveling theater show that day, and I had delivered a note to the office just that morning proving this to be true.

I said, *You made a mistake.* He said, *Computers don't make mistakes.* I said, *Your computer made a mistake.* He said, *You'll have to take it up with the principal.* I said, *Do you know that I hitchhike to school because I want to be here that badly?*

He didn't know what to do with me, what to say to me, I could see in his eyes what he was thinking: You don't belong here.

You don't belong.

I went back to my desk and sat long enough to feel something boil and freeze and shatter inside.

I would not beg to belong (certainly not on my knees).

Then I raised my hand and said, *I feel sick.*

The nurse called my mother. I knew she'd come. Me, sick! A dog whistle for her. A chance to play at mothering.

Once in the car I told her I wasn't really sick, even though my body ached underneath the pain I swallowed like Advil. Before the disappointment and frustration could settle onto her face, I followed up by saying that I wouldn't be going back to school.

I swear she smiled.

Thighs

Why didn't anyone take care of me?

Sometimes out of nowhere I'm hit with this question. Today it was post-climax. Sometimes pleasure holds pockets of grief.

I remember a winter night and my skinny fourteen-year-old thighs, shivering in the backseat of a car driven by someone old enough to buy booze, squeezed next to a man who was at least old enough to vote, his hands silently unbuttoning my jeans, fingers worming their way under cotton, finding warmth.

At least three other people sat in that car, all old enough to be there, one just next to the man with his fingers inside me. Their adult-sized thighs were touching.

I was high or drunk, but I remember feeling so alive. The December air whispering through the windows, cracked for the cigarette smoke. A pleasure I had only felt alone in my bedroom, under quilts, stuffed animals turned to look away from my curious and ashamed pleasure.

And then—why did he stop? Did someone tell him to? Did someone name my age?

Did someone try to take care of me?

Some part of me remembers an abrupt ending, and heat rising from my warmed thighs to my cheeks. And a longing for it to begin again. This secret touch felt better than what he did when he got me alone.

Did he feel shame? Or did I hold it for both of us?

Do I hold it for both of us?

By fourteen there was no parental voice that could find its way inside me. I had been parent to parents, to siblings, to myself for far too long to be able to take in and digest guidance or boundaries or punishment. I was untouchable, except for where I wanted to be touched.

I remember sitting with the woman who midwifed me into the world (she and I still share tea now and then). She knew this man who was *having sex to me*, as he put it. She told me, *He hates women.* She knew this because her adult daughter had dated him. In fact, the first night he fucked me, she had been with him at the party. He whispered to me that he would take her home and come back for me and my drug-addled barely teenaged body on a rough wool blanket spread on cool wet October grass. He said there was no need for protection when I asked, *I wouldn't do anything to you.*

The midwife tried to dissuade me from continuing on with this, with what I thought was true love. I remember her words sliding right off me, like I was made of smooth metal. A beloved acting teacher's words couldn't cling to me either, though I cried in her arms when he lied, when another woman answered his phone, when my heart tore like other parts had torn under his brief exploration (exploitation) of me.

But these well-meaning adults were talking to a child. Hoping that because I could moan and move like a grown adult, I was one, and could reason like one. I was not. I could not.

Why didn't anyone take care of me?

I've spent decades resolving the unresolvable. There is no good answer for this question. But there is this body.

This body that held my shame and his. This body which has become mine and mine alone. This body which has learned to be soothed. This body which no longer resides in a state of emergency, freezing like I did that winter. This body that can feel pleasure, and most times, the pleasure and shame are spread apart; they are no longer like thighs pressed together in the backseat of a full car.

My thighs sing to me:

I take care of me. I take care of me. I take care of me.

Skinny Baby

At eleven I was a skinny kid, but not skinny enough. Something told me that I was too big, even when I could clearly see the outline of my rib cage. I promised in my diary that I'd eat only lettuce—starting tomorrow—but not before one more candy bar.

Dear Diary, is Twix one candy bar? Or two?

The warm shame, mixed with caramel, chocolate, and wafers—all the stuff that hurt my teeth. I left the candy wrapper crumpled on the hardwood floor as I listened to the Doors on my record player. I sang along, sugar-high, *Baby, light my fire.*

I wanted to control something because I hadn't learned to lose control with booze just yet. That would come when I was thirteen. Keeping the starvation promises made me feel proud, like a parent. I wanted to be so small that I didn't exist at all, because it already felt that way to me. I felt like a winner when a cool girl, who I had a crush on, flashed her green eyes and hugged me through my thick green sweatshirt and said, *You are so tiny under there.*

My dad didn't eat when he was depressed or when his drinking was more excessive than usual. During those times he looked like a bone man, with slim blue jeans belted many holes deep. My mother ate until her stomach screamed. After a binge, she looked like shame only recognized in hindsight. Her blue jeans unbuttoned and folded over under her oversized t-shirts. I didn't like the feeling of being full, I wanted to be a bone man too, but I looked like shame all the same.

When my size zero blue jeans felt too tight, I refused to go up a size. I just starved myself back to zero instead.

I got better at control, and when my clavicle was clearly stated and my hip bones were like little knives, my dad would hand me a beer and say, *You got my genes, half-pint. Skinny just like me.* My mother said, *At least I won't have to pick up your crumpled candy wrappers anymore.* I wished my parents would pick me up and hold me like a skinny baby, whispering, *It's okay. It's okay. You belong to us.*

I was never sent to a hospital and given a tube to force-feed me like a goose. There were no grown-ups to say enough is enough. I was okay, I didn't lose my hair or my monthly bleed until I was twenty-seven and living in LA. That was the worst my disordered eating ever got. I was emaciated enough to get worried words from friends and to be scouted by a modeling agent. That business rewards kids who have the skill of deprivation. Eventually I found myself crumpled on my studio apartment's hardwood floor, too weak to make it to my bed. That's when I flipped open my flip phone and called someone to say, *I need you to know.* I said *anorexic* out loud.

After that overdue call for help, I couldn't stuff the truth back into my mouth. I couldn't eat those words like lettuce or candy or shame. I had to stop my starving. My self-denial trophies had to be turned in or melted down to make a cornucopia to fill with food. I learned how to eat, even during a breakup or a period of depression.

I learned to eat pizza, salads with croutons and creamy dressing full of fat, baked potatoes slathered with sour cream, corn on the cob dripping with butter, big plates of pasta with red sauce, fluffy rolls, Chinese noodles, Thai noodles, and Japanese noodles. I learned to eat whatever I wanted. I was shameless in nourishing my body.

I didn't know that soon I'd have to fight to keep weight on, not off. I didn't know that I wouldn't always be able to eat whatever I wanted, or that I would grieve each time another safe food was crossed off the list. I didn't know how my body would ache when I made a meal mistake, grain equals pain, or about the digests of diets I would try to digest. I didn't know that I would have to learn to eat again and again and again.

In seeking solutions to the painful problem of food, I tried white diets, simple diets, meat diets, broth diets, raw diets, keto diets, paleo diets, soup diets, fasting diets, vegan diets, warm diets, ayurvedic diets, smoothie diets, and Chinese medicine diets. Once my nephew, at eight years old, said, *Jess is on the no-food diet*. He wasn't far off, and his adorable accuracy gave me a good (almost empty) belly laugh.

My dad died before my digests of diets began. Though he too had bouts of anorexia and even told me so in the last months of his life, he loved food. Toward the end of his life, he could no longer eat food, not even soup. He received his nourishment through a feeding tube. The loss was devastating for him. One of my least favorite memories is how thoughtless I was to eat a stromboli in his hospital room. Mid-bite, I saw him watching me from his bed, with eyes hungry as a wolf and sad as a dying man. I boxed it back up, feeling guilty, and offered him a foot massage. My dad lost the ability to talk toward the end, and he loved to talk as much as he loved to eat. The cancer, grown from alcohol and cigarettes, required multiple surgeries, which robbed him of his Texas-tinted voice. Somehow, he still apologized to me for not being the dad I needed. As he struggled to speak with ravaged vocal cords, his tears left tiny circles on his thin green t-shirt. He turned into a real bone man. He was so thin that I was able to pick him up and hold him like a skinny baby, whispering, *It's okay, it's okay. You can go whenever you like.* My dad's genes, the alcoholic ones, killed him. But I survived.

My mother, who keeps hens as pets and doesn't eat meat, learned to make chicken soup for visits when that was all I could digest. Once when I was too sick to fly home to LA, my mother found me crying, in too much pain to move. She picked my crumpled tissues up off the floor and held me like a skinny baby, whispering, *It's okay, it's okay.*

Stay as long as you like. My tears left circles on the green flannel bed-sheets in the guest room, where my mother brought me bouquets of flowers and bowls of soup.

I broke up with food and took it back again too many times to count. I kept trying, but when food feels unsafe, it's easy for bones to start to become more defined. And since my body dysmorphia began at such a young age, my relationship with the weight loss was con-fusing. I had to go to battle with my perception of my reflection in the mirror. Eventually, I had to say the word *orthorexia* out loud. An obsession with only eating what I deemed to be healthy food was just as disordered as not eating at all. I had to keep telling the truth.

I take medications that make me dizzy and nauseous and steal all semblance of an appetite. I eat anyway. I miss popcorn and pasta and pizza, but I've learned to miss these things with grace. I've heard, *That must be so hard,* and *Corn is a grain?,* and *Have you tried...* over and over again. With a friendly smile, I answer, *I'm used to it!* and *It sure is!* and *Probably!* over and over again. I'm rarely invited to dinner parties, but I like dance parties better anyway. I swipe left on people with "foodie" in their bios and eat at home before dinner dates. I prefer to eat at out-door restaurants these days, because the pandemic isn't over for those of us with autoimmune diseases.

I was incredibly cautious, but Covid-19 finally caught me in the summer of 2022. I lost my taste and smell, and it still comes and goes without warning. It's weird but doesn't matter that much to me. At this point, food has lost most emotional flavors and is just a neces-sary ingredient for sustaining life, and something worthy of respect. Covid-19 also caused a major setback for my gastrointestinal issues and widespread body pain, and it seems to have launched me into perimenopause. I didn't get my period for two months after contract-ing that vascular virus. Then started the hot flashes, sleep issues, anx-iety, loss of sex drive, and a host of other hormonal symptoms. For something that some people have called *just a flu,* Covid-19 has had a major effect on my health, and therefore on my continued navigation of pain and food.

I have found foods that don't hurt my body, and I'm mostly consistent with the diet that works for me. Sometimes I get sad or bored and eat things that burn my gut and swell my joints, but I practice self-forgiveness, self-compassion, and as much self-restraint as I can muster. I do my very best to keep weight on. I want to exist. Most of the time I feel like a winner these days.

The beginning of my forties has found me skinny all over again, but not intentionally so. One recent afternoon as I dressed to meet a friend, I glanced in the mirror and my bone-man frame struck me as troublesome. Seeing the hollow of my cheeks and the slim of my limbs didn't light my fire the way it used to. What I saw registered as much too skinny, because now I could see my reflection without a dysmorphic view. I learned to respect food and the life it gives to me. As I gazed at my clavicle and hips, I thought, *This is called recovery.* And I beamed, like a proud parent, my skinny baby all grown up.

Eating Animals

I had a dead chicken in my hands. Robbed of its feathers, and head-less. I was washing it in the kitchen sink, my tears mixing with the tap water as they landed on the bird's goosebumped back. I was imagining my cats' bodies, skinned and being prepped for a pot of boiling water. This didn't feel that different to me. I was praying *thank you for your life, thank you for dying so that I can live.* It was some kind of holy horror cooking show. I would boil this once living creature, clean its carcass of meat, blend its cartilage, organs, and skin in my Vitamix, and make a broth of its bones. I would set aside the wishbone for childhood nos-talgia's sake. I would not ask the boyfriend, who would not put a ring on it, to break it in two with me, so the one with a bigger half could make a wish. He and I would later break in two, eleven years turned as dry as the saved pile of wishbones I threw away when I moved out of our condo.

I didn't want to eat animals. You can watch the torture they endure, in their pens, in their cages. The black-and-white undercover videos of factory farming are but a click away. Even the "lucky" ones, who graze and peck in green pastures, are born for slaughter. A beautiful death row with a monstrously quick turnaround, and no chance of a last-minute call from the governor granting clemency. I didn't want to eat animals or be any part of the industry that has no concern for sen-tience or suffering. Alas, the betrayal of twisted swollen intestines and a belly bloated to the size of *when are you expecting,* triggered by most everything I ate, shifted my ethical landscape. I had run out of options for sustenance, and at the urging of a trusted source, I found myself in the kitchen, my hands full of death. Death that would nourish, and maybe heal me.

I needed some nourishment and healing. I needed to eat. My diet had been shrinking, as I tried in vain to find the foods that wouldn't hurt. Everything tasted like pain and grief, or maybe worse, guilt when I gave into my cravings and found myself urgent-care bound. Blame, blame, blame showering down from my brain. *This is your fault.* Food was a punishment, restricted or not. My dreams were of feasts I could eat. I woke up, the taste of my slumber meals almost on my tongue, hungry and fearful of another day with the problem of food. I did not want the solution to be made of meat, but some wishes do not come true. Plant-based diets and wedding bells are not always meant to be.

I did my best to soften the blow of this solution. Pasture-raised. The butcher shop smelled of blood, and handsome tattooed and mustached men in white aprons with handfuls of red and pale pink called out numbers. The chicken I bought had a sign that told me what farm it had once called home. That made it better and worse. What I carried to my car inside a brown paper bag, stamped with a picture of a cow (I find it strange when the meat we eat is decorated with the animal it once was), felt illegal. The drive home, solemn.

After the sink-side tears and prayers, into a tall silver pot goes my country-side fowl. Carrots, celery, onions, olive oil, salt. Boil, then to a simmer. As the meaty steam filled the air of the condo, I wandered the carpeted floors, a wailing soldier, knowing the victory would not be mine. Once the job was complete, the war lost without honor or grace, I swallowed spoonfuls of Silly Putty–colored cartilage paté, as I had been told to do by the people who prescribed this gut healing regimen. I drank cups and cups of yellow broth, ate the boiled-onion-flavored meat. Between swallows and bites, I panicked and cried and complained. Did this crying and eating go on for days or for hours?

Long enough, anyway, for the five-star general of the home to grow impatient and cold. I was met with rolling eyes and sentences made of single words, sharp silence, and sighs. *Dramatic. Exhausting. Negative.*

I can see how those may have been the descriptors easiest to toss my way. It would have been heavier, harder to put arms around my suffering, offer a soft silence and murmurings of comfort. I heard and believed stories that I was hard to love, that I shrugged kindness off. I could not carry the heavy weight of his lacking empathy, and so I carried myself, best I could. I whispered words meant for a sorrowful child into my own ears as I acclimated to my new life as a carnivore, letting go my attachment to an identity that was starving me in its compassion and care for other living things.

Learning to eat death proved to be well worth the sorrow. I grew stronger, and much to my once vegan mind's disappointment, the gut-healing power of sentient beings was made clear. I had to eat the judgment I once held for the carnivorous crowd right along with the baked beef and homemade cultured cream. The act of ingesting what I had denied myself delivered old grief and new love. The places where I had lacked empathy and understanding were tenderized. Those mallets of humility find me every time.

I think that to heal is to be humbled. I had to see how I pushed love away. How I settled for what I told myself was enough. How I starved. Seeing my starving meant feeling, and feeling meant changing, and changing meant healing. As the lining of my stomach was soothed by the warm broth and soft meat, my humbled heart no longer wanted to be wishbone-dry, torn in two. I had no diamond on my finger, but I sparkled all the same, and the future found me whole, glistening, and alive.

The broth of bones and hand-shaped hamburgers released me from the bloating and burning bowels. My face, acne prone since I became a "true friend of animals" many years before, cleared. My nails, brittle from biting, grew thick and strong. I could not deny my body's wisdom, so obviously displayed. Healing had transpired. Heal your gut, heal your life. I still often wish that plants could be my medicine. I still find wisps of wishes for a love that could only survive if I let my sparkle die, but I stopped wishing so I could start living.

For me, eating animals is what I imagine it might be like to scale a mountain, with no safety lines (*dramatic* indeed). You must not think about anything but the very moment you are existing in, lest you remember what you are doing and take a long fall to the jagged ground. I do not think about what I am eating when I eat animals. I do not think of their sweet, sad eyes, or how they want to live just as I do. I could not carry on this way if I did. I wash and whisper prayers of gratitude to what was once whole, glistening, and alive, and then I call it food. I call it love. I call it a life for a life. You are what you eat and I am alive.

Addiction: The Disease of Post-Trauma

Alcohol was my best friend. I needed that friend to hold my hand while the storms of trauma raged inside my developing mind and ravaged my young body. Our friendship started when I was twelve, and from age fourteen to age twenty-seven I was never without it for more than a month. Like any good best friend, it offered comfort when sadness overtook me, gave me courage when I couldn't work up the nerve to tell a pretty girl I liked her, lifted the heavy curtains of boredom when entertainment was sparse, helped me forget when shame wrapped me in its gray embrace, and made me feel like I was enough when the ghosts of my childhood whispered that I would never be. Alcohol wasn't my only friend—there were others that helped me get by—but it was the one who had the other half of the heart pendant that hung on a chain just below my clavicle.

I was loyal to my best friend until I started to recognize the way it couldn't always be trusted to want what was best for me, how it would leave me alone in drunken darkness with strange men, the pangs of depression and anxiety it would wake me with each morning, and perhaps the worst thing, when it simply ceased to flip the switch of intoxication and left me draining bottles empty, and begging for the relief it once offered.

Eventually I had to give up my best friend. Our friendship, once the medicine that treated the painful imprints of my past, became toxic. That poisoned partnership needed to be severed permanently, lest it drag me down into a slow bad death or take me out in a sudden crash of steel on steel after telling me I was fine to drive. We said our last goodbye on a hotel rooftop in Miami. I watched my once bosom buddy, my BFF, fall the twenty stories to the concrete below, shattering like an empty bottle. The glittering shards as small as fine soft grains of sand.

But before all that, I was an infant high on cocaine. My mother was just a kid, and she wasn't thinking of the consequences when she partook and then nursed me. She wasn't even the hard drug type, but something came over her, or grew up under her, and into her nose went the white lines. For reasons unknown, she told me about this mistake with great remorse when I was fourteen. I was a speedy baby, too small to run off the high. I shook all night, so the story goes. My mother's mistake that night wasn't made with malice. She may not have been considering that I might be harmed. My first experience with drugs was an accident. Later in life, I would grow to love cocaine, but I had the discipline to stay away from it, for the most part.

Because of my undiagnosed ADHD, chronic fatigue, and rebellion against my mother's wishes, I intentionally picked up my next drug before I was ten. Caffeine. It was a good friend to me from the beginning, giving me the focus and energy I lacked. I used to take shots of Jolt Cola with my friends at the party house in Prospect Park my dad would take us to. We lined up shot glasses, just like the adults did, and poured from the glass bottle of legal speed.

One night at that same house, we kids found ourselves alone for such a long time that we went hunting for our parents. We found them in a third-floor bathroom, piled together against black and white tiles, legs and arms akimbo. They were smoking pot and becoming "blood brothers." Blood on their thumbs and lips, from sucking on the cuts they had rubbed together. Wide red eyes and smiles. *Come innnnnn here*, they moaned with thick laughter in their throats. We backed out, an accordion of small bodies, folding up and then scattering back down the two flights of wide wooden steps to the kitchen, falling into chairs with frightened giggles. Going in for another round of shots, when highly caffeinated soda was enough to get us high.

When I was a teenager and soon to be kicked out of my mother's house for doing drugs and having sex and being immune to any rules, she acknowledged my predicament. Said something like, *I treated you like an adult and now you won't act like a child. I guess that's my fault.* It was a moment of such truth and accountability, but in the end, it didn't stop her from sending me away for my misdeeds. I imagine she tried her best to keep me close, but her tools were seriously limited, and I was, as Axl Rose my adolescent obsession sang, "on a night train, ready to crash and burn." I've often wondered if I would be better off, or worse, if she had tossed me into rehab instead of out of the house.

Ultimately, I never needed to go to rehab, but it's funny how my oldest addiction is still with me. I have never given up caffeine, except for brief stints at fourteen and thirty, when controlling boyfriends tried to make me quit. I didn't last long, and I think my uncaffeinated mood was jarring enough to throw both off their high stimulant-free horses. I love caffeine. However, my cup of coffee in the morning, or my tea or diet soda in the afternoon, is a far cry from what I did as a teenage alcoholic.

I would work until 9 at night, and then as long as I didn't work my second job the next day, I would drink until 3 a.m. I had to be at work at 3 p.m., so I'd wake up at 11 and take two caffeine pills and two Advil. Then back to bed for an hour. I'd wake up hangoverless and ready to take on the day. Once at work, I'd start with a cup of coffee. That was followed by a Mountain Dew, and often another coffee from the café across from the restaurant, this one with a few shots of espresso added. I also became a fan of Red Bull on one of the family road trips to Florida with my dad. You could only get them at truck stops back then. I bounced in the back of the car, pinball style. Ecstatic, until the crash.

At twelve I started smoking cigarettes. I planned to get this habit going. Set an alarm for midnight, knowing my dad would be too drunk to wake to it. Then I silently swiped one of his Marlboro Reds and smoked it in the bathroom.

When I was officially a teenager, I added in cannabis, once writing a letter to *Teen* magazine shaming them for calling this magical plant a gateway drug. I'm glad they didn't print it, because I would have had to tear out the page and eat it. By fourteen I had done a fair amount of LSD and psilocybin, and tried meth once and crack a few times. And let's not leave out pharmaceuticals. After a house fire that we narrowly escaped, in which our neighbors died despite my mother and I trying to save them, a friend of the family gave me a Xanax. What a miracle. The way everything was suddenly okay, much like the first time I got drunk. Breath, relaxation, peace of mind.

Controlling boyfriend number one showed up around the time I started experimenting with hard drugs. By the time he started threatening to kill himself if I so much as smoked a cigarette, I was already firmly under his thumb. His behavior was textbook antisocial personality disorder, and the abuse I experienced reflected that likely diagnosis to a tee. He would scream at me if a man on the street noticed me. He isolated me from my friends and family, constantly accused me of cheating on him, and would keep me trapped in a room with him until I agreed with whatever terrible things he was saying about me. A sadist, he liked to get me in his car in the boiling East Coast summer, roll up the windows, turn off the AC, and wait until I was pouring sweat and begging for air. I once wrote in a journal that I would let him fuck my face just so he would stop berating me and let me go to sleep. He never once made me cum. Even with all that, it took a miracle for me to leave him. I was just as addicted to him as I have ever been to any drug.

I think it's a miracle that I never got hooked on hard drugs, not that alcohol isn't a hard drug. It's culturally accepted and even expected, but over 140,000 people die *every year* in the US due to excessive consumption of alcohol, and around 10,000 people are killed by drunk drivers.[1] Heroin-related overdoses, on the other hand, kill about the same amount of people in the US over the span of *twenty years*.[2] (Who's hard now, heroin?) Alcohol killed my dad, my dad's mom, nearly killed another family member due to several suicide attempts while drunk, likely killed my maternal great-great-grandfather, and may yet kill a few other relatives who are drinking like tomorrow will never come. Some people don't know when a friendship has turned deadly, or even if they know, they just can't seem to let it fall from the roof and shatter. Alcohol didn't kill me, and one day at a time, it never will.

I've been in recovery and alcohol-free since 2007. Of my fourteen years of drinking, I was only of legal drinking age for half of them. I've now been sober for longer than I drank. When I stopped drinking, I was barely drinking. It didn't make me feel free anymore, and the negative consequences made it hard to breathe easy. At thirteen, the substance had been the best friend of my dreams. I *needed* an escape from the reality of my life and the toll it took on my mental health. The effects of trauma were dampened, and the shame and self-loathing I carried lessened. Drinking also dulled the physical pain that walked with me from such a young age. The headaches and stomachaches, relieved temporarily. Much like that controlling and abusive boyfriend, alcohol may have saved my life, but also hurt me deeply.

I was told from a very young age that if I drank, I'd be *just like my dad*—and after I started drinking, I was screamed at: *You little asshole, you're going to end up a fucking alcoholic, just like him.* The message being that casual and responsible drinking was not possible for me because

I was genetically predisposed to be an alcoholic. Even so, I was never under any illusion that I wouldn't drink. As a teenager I would do thirty-day sober challenges to prove to myself that I wasn't an alcoholic. In my late teens and early twenties I would give myself talks in the bathroom mirror of bars (it was easy to be an underage drinker in the '90s, especially when you'd been playing an adult for many years) and parties once I was pleasantly drunk. I'd promise my happy reflection that I wouldn't have another drink. Those mirror talks were always a sure sign that I'd be back in the bathroom in a few hours, vomiting my guts out in the toilet. I became highly adept at throwing up without anyone ever knowing. I taught myself how to drink like a professional; the early alarm and caffeine pills were part of that skill set. There was a time around age seventeen when I got so good at drinking, I couldn't get drunk anymore. A fifth of vodka left me feeling a bit ragged but barely intoxicated.

My bottoming-out experience became less dramatic as I got older. Once my rock bottoms were getting tossed out of clubs with a bouncer holding each of my arms and swinging me out the door like they do in the movies, fucking other people's partners, and kneeling in alleys in the morning light, throwing up, while first-shift restaurant workers smoked cigarettes at the back door and watched. Later when I was trying with all my might to control my drinking, my rock bottoms were me alone in my studio apartment drinking Scotch and taking pills, wishing I had the courage to take the whole bottle. At that point, I only drank occasionally because I had begun to understand that I *was* becoming my dad. I didn't want anyone to see what I was becoming. A lonely binge now and then, a rationing of the medicine that had once helped me live, not replaced with anything but isolation, white knuckles, and shame. I relapsed into anorexic behavior, my hair falling out and my period stopping. I thought about killing myself every day. My best friend had turned on me. Drinking didn't feel like an option anymore, but not drinking didn't feel like an option either. How to live?

Was the prophecy of my "alcoholism" made true by the idea being violently injected into my developing mind? Would I have landed there without the trials and tribulations of my early life? Is alcoholism a disease, or as an old friend and mentor, Tracy McMillan, once said to me, is alcohol abuse a symptom of *the disease of post-trauma*? Studies on adverse childhood experiences (ACEs) and substance dependence seem to back up this theory, along with explaining the cause of numerous chronic conditions.[3]

There are a plethora of studies on how bad a bad childhood is for humans. The toxic stress of an adverse childhood can negatively impact your physical and mental health, leading to lifelong chronic conditions. It's been shown that ACEs can interfere with brain development and affect the way your nervous system responds to adversity and stress.[4] Around 61 percent of adults in the US have at least one ACE, and approximately 16 percent have at least four.[5] People with ACEs are more likely to be smokers and to keep smoking even when there are health consequences.[6] ACEs increase the risk of chronic obstructive pulmonary disease, and that's not just for smokers.[7] The risk of dyslipidemia, chronic lung disease, asthma, liver disease, digestive disease, kidney disease, arthritis, and additional chronic diseases shoots up for those with at least four ACEs.[8] The possibility of suicide is *thirty times* more likely if you have four or more ACEs.[9] With an ACE score of 6 or more, your lifespan could be shortened by *twenty years.*[10] LGBTQ+ kids, girls, and underrecognized and historically excluded and disinvested groups of youth may have an increased risk of having four or more ACEs.[11] Studies have suggested that ACEs can lead to fibromyalgia, heart disease, diabetes, autoimmune diseases, depression, anxiety, poverty, and the list goes on.[12] In short having a fucked-up childhood is not good for your health and well-being.[13] My ACE score is 7.

No matter your ACE score, here's some good news: Adverse childhood experiences are not set in stone. Your ACE survey doesn't account for positive childhood experiences (PCEs) that might decrease the negative effects.[14] Just one trusted adult can increase resilience and lower the impact of adverse experiences.[15] Greater family connection can lead to greater flourishing in adulthood, even when there are ACEs involved.[16] Psychotherapy in childhood has been shown to reduce psychopathological symptoms.[17] Your fate is not sealed by what happened to you—even glimmers of goodness can change your trajectory.

We had a neighbor when I was five or six who had long thick messy braids and the most warm and welcoming smile. I remember sitting at her kitchen bar on a stool while she poured me some juice and talked to me. I felt safe and seen. The brief time I knew her still resonates in my heart.

There was a private progressive school that my mother had attended as a kid, and where she had a part-time cleaning job when I was little. I often went with her and played in the playground, and watched my younger sisters, while I waited for my mother to be done. One of the first-grade teachers thought I was a bright and curious child and would be a good addition to her class, but my mother couldn't afford the expensive tuition. That teacher went to the heads of the school and advocated for me to be able to go for free. They didn't allow it, but the fact that she did that for me was incredibly meaningful. When I eventually went to that school later on, my teachers provided a positive childhood experience. One special teacher once told me that if she had a kid, she wished they would be just like me. She made me feel like I was deserving of that kind of love. She taught me to treat others with kindness (being bullied at home, I was a bit of a bully for a short period). She cast me in my first leading role in a play, and when I was terrified and said no, she lovingly convinced me. I've been an actor ever since. She encouraged my writing and stuck up for me when another teacher was treating me badly.

The two men who owned a restaurant I worked at (the one I took caffeine pills for) offered me not only a job but stability, accountability, and a fatherly sort of love. The dad of one of my teenage boyfriends basically wanted to adopt me. A family who briefly took me in at fourteen treated me as one of their own. A woman who was a friend of my dad's was a confidant and caretaker. I also had a few therapists before I turned eighteen who tried to help me make sense of what I was going through.

I had an aunt and uncle who offered a safe and welcoming environment to visit. My uncle introduced me to Nirvana and the Pixies while kids my age were listening to New Kids on the Block. He was also an artist and would take specific requests for cartoon-style drawings— like "a dog holding a balloon at a picnic birthday party where the cake almost falls over"—done with brightly colored high-quality markers. My aunt told hilarious stories that made me laugh so hard it hurt and I had to beg her to stop. She was a dancer and took me to see modern dance in the city and then to fancy dinners afterward. They both listened to me and made life seem magical.

My maternal grandmother, while she had her issues (and had horribly abused my mother), was mostly loving to me. I loved to fall asleep in her bed when I slept over. She would stroke my head and say sweet things that I never really heard because I drifted off so quickly. She paid for things like piano lessons and taught me to ride a horse as soon as I was big enough to sit on the saddle and hold the reins. My maternal grandfather was probably the closest thing to a *real* adult I had as a kid. He treated me like a kid and expected me to behave like one. While I didn't listen or obey, he made his opinions known and didn't let up. He didn't give up on me, even when I was too far gone to reach. He couldn't rein me in, like I had learned to do with their horses, but the fact that he kept trying was such an act of love.

And there was my mother reading me endless children's books, calling me Jessica Rose with ten pink toes and then kissing me all over my face, scratching my back, letting me climb on her back while pretending to be the turtle from *The NeverEnding Story* and sneezing me off, singing me to sleep (*like a ship in the harbor, like a mother and child, like a light in the darkness, I'll hold you a while...*), making fried tofu cut into the shape of a bunny with a cookie cutter, prioritizing nature and art, teaching me to be sex-positive and that it was totally okay to be bisexual, buying me my first computer when I was sixteen (a huge purchase, especially for a kid she was estranged from!), doing her best every day to break the generational curse of ACEs, failing often, but always trying again. Some of my worst ACEs came from her, but also some of my best PCEs.

And my dad caused a good number of my ACEs, but he loved me fiercely. He filled my life with many rich and exciting experiences. He gave me a deep love of film and music. He introduced me to the great filmmakers and actors of his time. He took me to see Paul McCartney and Wings when I was eight and once waited in line overnight to get me front-row tickets to see Tori Amos. He was playful and fun, never tiring from games of playground monster or freeze tag. He was proud of me and expressed it every chance he got. He taught me not to trust the cops and that Black people had it the worst because of systemic racism. He taught me that Palestine should be free and that abortion is healthcare. He taught me to cover my drink and how to pay attention to subtle danger cues from men. Although when it came down to it, he couldn't stay alive for me, he would have died for me without a second thought.

I imagine that it was all these PCEs that have kept me sober from alcohol for all these years, and even allowed me to quit drinking in the first place. These glimmers of goodness are most likely what brought me back from the literal edge, multiple times. The fact that I had supportive adults, albeit inconsistently or for short periods, has given me the resilience to stay here and continue to grow. We are not all so lucky. I count my blessings. Trauma can seep deep into our DNA, twisting and contorting the genes that dictate how our bodies respond to stress and hardship, like adverse childhood experiences.

Exposure to trauma has been shown to cause changes at the molecular level, altering the very expression of our genes. And these changes can be passed down to future generations, etched into the fabric of our DNA. The gift that keeps giving. One study explored the epigenetic changes present in Holocaust survivors and their offspring. Both generations showed striking changes in the genes responsible for regulating our body's response to stress.[18] Another, and evidently less flawed study, delved into the paternal children of those who were in the Civil War, with similar results.[19] A study from 2020 suggests that transatlantic enslavement trade has a genetic impact on Black Americans today.[20] Science continues to offer visceral reminders of how far-reaching the imprint of trauma may be.

For me, the findings of these scientific explorations help release shame and blame. Knowing that I was most likely wired for addictive behaviors and a rough ride from before birth makes self-compassion and forgiveness abundant and accessible. This information also steers me away from blaming my parents for my adverse childhood and the negative consequences. The science of epigenetics says that perhaps their DNA was marked before birth too, and their parents before them. We are in this together. We do our best to lessen the imprint on the next generation. We fail, but perhaps not as badly as our predecessors. We do our best to move as quickly as we can, sometimes shocked by the new territory we are given access to when we change the direction of the sail even a few degrees. A new continent, a new landscape, and a new way to live. For me that new life has freed me from my addictive behaviors with alcohol.

Addiction limits our ability to evolve psychologically and spiri-tually. That can be addiction of any kind, from the seemingly trivial (our phones being no exception) to the kind that leaves you on the streets and down to ninety-eight pounds with rotting teeth within a year. I needed to stop drinking before I could set sail to a new world. Of course, I was able to evolve even when I was drinking; if I hadn't evolved, I never would have been able to quit.

I accepted that alcohol could no longer be my best friend the night I was on top of that tall hotel in Miami. The thick air felt strong enough to pick me up and hold me. I had been flown there and was being put up because I was the lead in a film screening at a film festival. I should have been over the moon with excitement and joy; instead I was contemplating testing that thick night air by taking a leap off the roof. I had been surrounded by free alcohol all night—there may have even been a vodka fountain of some kind. My hands hurt from how white my knuckles were. I had been supplementing with over-the-counter cold medicine, but it wasn't cutting it. I hadn't drank, but now I wanted to die. I didn't want to drink, but I didn't know how to live with all the pain that had rushed to the surface when I tried to stop for good. I couldn't live with alcohol and I couldn't live without it.

I can only call it a moment of grace that I picked up the phone that night. I talked to someone who had been sober for years. He talked me off the edge, and into an AA meeting. That was the beginning of a new chapter that has been followed by many more. It's not always pretty and it's far from perfect, but I continue to evolve. I continue to live, and often I live well. Would I have had that moment of grace if not for the neighbor with the warm smile and apple juice, without the teachers who saw me and loved me, without the turtle sneezes and the bunny-shaped tofu, without the flawed but fierce love? Perhaps not.

The day after that Miami rooftop experience, I swam in the sea. It was glittering, clear and blue, the fine grains of sand soft as silk under my feet. The beautiful people on the beach, scantily clad with jewel-toned thongs and mesh tops, didn't know that I was in the ocean seeing a new continent within swimming distance. I swam and swam. I found shore and then kept swimming. I keep swimming, taking deep breaths and diving for treasures in the places that still hurt, finding beauty in the pain. There have been many new lands to explore since that night, that choice that wasn't really a choice but rather a divine gift that I cannot explain. I find myself on the surface of the water, in the deepest depths, and on every shore. I continue to find yet another unknown layer I thought I knew, to offer healing to. Each time I feel the shaking baby inside me, I love them more fiercely, as I sing, *like a ship in the harbor*, more sweetly.

I have found new best friends in kind and loving humans and community, in my tiny scruffy dog, in myself, and in the many forms of God. These friends are true and deserve my loyalty. They offer medicine that heals instead of hurts. This is the kind of friendship that can challenge my very DNA and make me a person who lessens the imprints of generational trauma on the newest members of my family line. Maybe with friends like these, the disease of post-trauma doesn't stand a chance.

The List

Sunshine afternoon. I'm three years old, on my own, with my friend and her older brothers and boy cousins, behind a big wooden shed with holes in the roof next to the skinny white house where I live with my still-in-love parents and my baby sister who was my belated birthday present when I was two years old. One of the boys asks, *Do you dare me?*

Moonlit middle of the night. I'm fourteen years old, on my own, with a nineteen-year-old man who looks like he is twenty-five, behind tall dry grass naked on a scratchy wool blanket in the field next to the big old house where I live with stepbrothers who never have to wash the dishes or clean the toilet bowls. The man whispers, *I would never do anything bad to you.*

Gray and cloudy late afternoon. I'm fifteen years old, on my own, surrounded by doctors and four interns, who *I* did not invite to stay, behind a thin and creased paper gown, pushed up to my waist, next to the shiny metal tray where tiny slices of cervix are housed in plastic test tubes marked with my name. A nameless doctor insists, *You won't need anything stronger, Advil will be fine.*

Purple-skied evening. I'm thirty-two years old, on my own, on my back, head off the edge of the bed, with the cock of a then trusted man in my mouth, behind the walls of love bombs and gaslights that have been erected around me, next to an unlocked door that I just can't seem to open and walk out through. He says nothing, *asks* nothing, a mask-slipped smile, a punishment, my shocked mouth fills with piss.

Deep night with waves-on-cliff sounds. I'm thirty-seven years old, on my own, with a powerful man who groomed me like a pretty pony for a week, behind his high-thread-count top sheet, but also frozen, next to myself watching his wrinkled and age-spotted hands move higher up thighs I could swear are mine as he gives me a *friendly* massage. I come back to my body, I say *No*, I put my clothes back on and move hastily to the door, he whimpers, *But my wife won't do this with me.*

This is *the list* that I lay beside lists of the one in three vulva-bearing humans. (I don't discount the one in six men, boys, and people with penises. I see you.) And the list is longer if I include the many times I didn't say no but surely didn't say yes. A young man, addicted to filling his arms with heroin, spitting in my face repeatedly in his parents' attic. Covert emotional abuse and subtle coercive control disguised as BDSM. Shredding my knees and elbows while dragging myself across a carpet to get away from a man who wanted to switch his uninvited sharp-fingernail fingers in my unlubed ass with his long veiny dick. Unwittingly playing a sleeping beauty sex doll for someone who *just wanted to watch me sleep.* The face fuckings too fast to decline. All the times I was far too drunk to come close to consenting.

The list has lived in my lining and labia. It's been woven into the web of root-level muscles. It has stagnated in the bowl of my pelvis. *The list* has poured into my throat, choked me, voiceless and sore. It's been shoved in my anus, fissures and hemorrhoids, vagus disruption, body dysfunction. I am not alone. So many carry *the list* of exploitation and violation in places meant for pleasure, imprinting the sensitive and tender spots with grief and shame. We hold subtle and explicit horrors inside the beauty of our bodies. Our bodies can't be forcefully quieted as our voices may have been, and they bellow out, *Believe me, believe me, believe me.*

This bellowing call to belief, to recognition, to recovery and resolution, can so often come in the form of pain. I have lived with the pain of sexual violation, and I have learned to listen to it as the wisdom of my body. I count myself lucky that my pain rarely manifests itself as shame. I know how very privileged I am to be nearly shameless about my sexuality, in all its many expressions over the years. I never saw sex as something to be ashamed of. My parents did a beautiful job of creating mostly sex-positive households. There *was* an ocean of emotional incest, which left its water stains, but rarely have those marks been shame shaped. And yet, some percentage of my past and present chronic physical and emotional pain can be explained by *the list*.

My body exposed this explanation in a multitude of ways. Another kind of list.

The tears of grief that used to spontaneously burst forth with every self-produced climax in solitude. Different from the kind of ecstatic sobbing that soaks beds after seeing God during sex, solo or otherwise. Or the joyful weeping that winds around a single body or more, a song of satisfaction and delight. This was something else. Heavy, but hollow. Desperate, but resigned. Those tears were the bellow of my body.

The mystery sore throats and loss of my voice. The sudden and strange hemorrhoids that sent me to urgent care when the pain left me unable to work. The lesions inside my bladder, shown by a tiny camera slid into my sore urethra and urinary tract (that procedure itself was a traumatic event). My pelvic floor as hard and compacted as a concrete floor. The ache in my hips. My sweet psoas muscle, a spring squeezed tight. These were the bellow of my body.

Each of these pains is not made entirely of sexual trauma. Trauma of any kind will make the body bellow. And violations of the sexual kind show up in my bellyaches and headaches and heartaches too. The particular cries of my body, listed as a result of my list, just seem to have the sound of stolen *nos* at a higher volume than others. Knowing this allows me to lovingly attend to my bellowing body with understanding and clear intention.

That understanding and intentionality led me to a multitude of modalities and methods. Another kind of list.

Those grieving climax tears slowly faded. I couldn't credit it to any one thing, so I will say that the resolution of that salty subcortical flood of grief came gradually though all the modalities and methods. And then one day it became, *Oh, I used to cry when I came. I don't anymore.* Now my sex-soaked tears are all joyful or spirit-filled or just a simple release.

My throat has been more or less chronically sore since Covid-19 captured me just once. It was at a women's retreat, where I was the only one openly out of the binary, and where I fell in love with a woman but didn't kiss her beautiful face because that beautiful face graced wedding photos and the wedding wasn't mine. Before then, the stolen *no*s that made my throat hurt were returned though somatic trauma resolution, Fitzmaurice Voicework, learning to speak my truth, and sipping soothing warm drinks while saying sweet words to myself. It also helped greatly that, save the frozen seaside moment when I was thirty-seven, and a few small snags before that, I've learned to speak my *no* with a generous volume and not a shake in my voice.

The hemorrhoids. Oh the hemorrhoids. These are in big part due to the chronic constipation I've had since I was too tiny to properly fit on a toilet seat. That constipation the result of C-PTSD, and the chronic illnesses that grew out of that. The issues with my anus are also related to the list of sexual abuse and assault. Recently what was once only internal hemorrhoids and fissures quite literally popped out of my ass. That came right after a powerful energy work session focused on my root chakra, the place where sexual trauma is often held. It didn't matter that the session was via Zoom, it had a clear impact. That external hemorrhoid was a many-week ordeal that eventually found me in stirrups with a very nice woman in a white coat looking at my bulging asshole. I suppose it was a purging of sorts. A particularly painful purging that continues to flare up now and then and may require surgery. Internal anal and vaginal bodywork have been helpful in processing and releasing that stored trauma. The sitz bath has been a good friend of mine, as have witch hazel cotton pads.

After the hellish hemorrhoid, I have found steroid suppositories to be a godsend. I also abstain from anal sex with anything bigger than a finger, the nails trimmed and lube applied.

I'll pair together my inflamed bladder and urinary tract and the concrete muscles of my pelvic floor, as both were greatly improved though pelvic floor therapy. It started in a small low-lit room with a man who was a physical therapist that vulva owners celebrated in whispers. He worked only externally on me and always had a woman in the room to promote a sense of safety and consent. Then into a yurt with my friend, colleague, and practitioner, the vulva whisperer herself, Kimberly Ann Johnson. One session with her and my pee came out in a strong steady stream for the first time in years. It was temporary, but with more sessions there were lasting and permanent effects. She is also the one who I trusted enough to gently work on my rectum, and the one who told me that I needed animal protein in order to heal. She was right. I didn't stop with the pelvic floor work there. I knew there was more relief to be had and that deep layers of *the list* lived in that majestic web of muscles. I've had three other pelvic floor therapists, each one a gem of a human. That profession calls to a certain demographic. I've cried and laughed and gasped and sighed and yawned on their paper-covered tables. I've wiped lubricant and sometimes tears off with the tissues they leave by a small trash can. There were times I was so numb I couldn't feel their fingers. Times when even the lightest touch inside me on just the right spot felt like salt and lemon juice on an open wound. Times when warmth and aliveness spread into all the muscles, and I felt myself heal in real time. *The list* still makes that part of my body bellow every so often, but the layers are less and less.

The ache in my hips comes and goes, but the ache of *the list* has released from them. Hip openers on a yoga mat, held for long minutes in a warm room, and myofascial release can answer for this. As for my sweet psoas, understanding its messages was what unsprang that spring. Once understood, I attended to the freeze and uncompleted flight that had squeezed it so tight. Somatic trauma resolution, massage, relaxation, and stunningly simple exercises got the gold. I say stunningly simple because the pain I experienced before was so stunningly complex.

Listening to the bellows of my body that cried out about *the list* and responding to the list of pains with the list of modalities and methods, I created yet another kind of list.

I vow to never bypass my body's signals not to have sex with someone who isn't a match for me or who doesn't recognize and exclaim my value and worth as a human being.

I vow to listen to and honor the subtle flight and freeze cues of my nervous system.

I vow to advocate for my sexual health and demand the respect and care I deserve from medical professionals.

I vow to always speak my truth about my sexual pleasure, desires, and boundaries.

I vow to continue the limbic revision that allows feeling deeply safe to also be deeply sexy.

I vow to continue resolving any layers of sexual trauma that are revealed.

I vow to care for my body and give it the things it needs to thrive.

I vow to use *the list* to learn, grow, and help others.

I vow to be compassionate and kind to myself, remembering that healing isn't linear, and while perfection isn't possible, progress is.

I vow to love the three-year-old behind the shed, the fourteen-year-old behind the tall grass, the fifteen-year-old behind the paper gown, the thirty-two-year-old behind the walls, the thirty-seven-year-old behind the sheet.

I vow to show all parts of me how much better it can be.

Choose Me

I had been on a Dilaudid drip for five days and I wanted to have a baby. That's the drug that Nadine, played by Heather Graham, overdoses on in the classic Gus Van Sant film *Drugstore Cowboy*. When I was rolled into the ER, morphine did nothing to relieve my pain, so they gave me the good stuff, ten times stronger than morphine. Toward the end of my stay at the hospital, I suggested we take it down a notch and switch to morphine. The response was that I could stay on this drug or receive Tylenol only. I stuck with the Dilaudid.

I didn't know I had ulcers and extreme chronic gastritis until the pain was so bad I was ripped from a meditation retreat to spend almost a week in a hospital 400 miles from home. My stomach stopped bleeding, but I couldn't pee because I was so constipated from the drugs, lack of movement, and the gastrointestinal issues beyond what had led to the plastic band around my wrist. Having interstitial cystitis and an almost full bladder for days on end was physically alarming to say the least. Although the bleed had ceased and with it the rolling contractions of breathtaking pain that laughed in the face of mere morphine, it wasn't yet safe for me to leave.

My memory of that hospital stay is blurred and spotty. I was on so many drugs, including Ambien (that is some wild shit), and I had been in deep meditation for a few days before this whole adventure began. I have wisps of recollection. There were kind nurses, exhausted and distracted nurses, a gaslighting doctor who spoke about me as if I weren't in the room, and an overly nice doctor with a saccharine voice who was surrounded by eager-eyed residents. My aunt who lived in the area came by for visits, as did a friend who lived an hour away. I barely remember them being there. The most consistent fixture at my bedside was my then partner, who I had been on the meditation retreat with.

He went back and forth between sitting with me and being my health advocate and sitting on a meditation cushion in front of some monastics from the Thai Forest tradition. I don't actually know how often he left the hospital to meditate or left the monastery to caretake. What I do know is that the way he showed up and dealt with the doctors, tried to comfort me through agonizing pain and the fear of an emergency endoscopy, made sure I got the right medications, and at least a night or two slept in a chair next to my bed, led me to believe that he was finally going to be ready to tie the knot.

I had been asking for a few years already. When I wasn't stuffing my desire into my guts, that is. He said no the first time, and I told myself that I wouldn't be one of *those* people who break up just because their partner isn't ready to make it official in the eyes of the law. I was afraid that if I pushed the matter, I'd lose him. I silently vowed not to bring it up again for one year. It's humbling to think back to that version of me who was willing to bypass my truth out of fear of losing a relationship that didn't meet my needs. We were soaking in a hot tub when he gave me several reasons as to why he wasn't ready to marry me. Ways that I was not yet the right one to bet forever on. I let the steam, rising from the jet-fueled bubbling water, carry away my disappointment and feelings of rejection and set about to address the things that made me not yet marriage material according to him.

This happened again and again over the next eight years. The goalposts kept moving until I had *fixed* everything about myself that was flagged as an obstacle to commitment. Finally, all he could say was, *I want to get married and have kids, I'm just not sure I want it with you.* Still,

I stayed. I even convinced myself that it was understandable that he told me my chronic conditions were one of the reasons that he wasn't sure about me. It *is* understandable, but if that's how someone feels, I now believe that it's on them to leave the relationship and let the other person meet someone who can fully accept them as they are, multiple diagnoses and all. As excruciating as it was, I knew that I wouldn't leave until I was good and ready to leave. I gave myself grace and patience and worked to heal the parts of myself that were so attached (or you might say addicted) to someone who was unable to choose me or really even see me.

I had never really been that marriage focused. I *never* had fantasies about wearing white or floral table arrangements. I was engaged once, but it was to a woman before we had marriage equality in the US, and we broke up before human rights won out (how disturbing that those rights are now one SCOTUS ruling from being taken away). But I wanted to marry this guy and I had known it from very early on. I saw our future laid out in front of us. Partners in life and art. Parents who would raise a cool kid. I wanted to create a home full of love, spirituality, and creativity.

Nice fantasy, but that was never going to happen, even if he did marry me. It looked great on the outside, but the relationship was rotten to the core. Bringing a child into that relationship would have been a grave mistake. Yet I was married to denial, committed to avoiding the truth of my situation. I unconsciously reasoned that if I didn't let myself fully see and take in the dysfunction of the relationship and the mistreatment I was experiencing, then I didn't have to feel the despair and grief that was just below the surface.

This perfectly mirrored the much-needed coping mechanisms of my childhood. As a kid, fantasy and denial helped me survive neglect and abuse. Without that escape, reality would have been too much to bear. The problem is that I brought that once-necessary coping mechanism into my adult life and it kept me stuck in a relationship that was generally unsatisfying at best, and emotionally, physically, and spiritually devastating at worst.

My body knew the score from the very beginning of that relationship. I started having frequent migraines and kidney infections a few months in. I also experienced a sharp increase in my complex PTSD (C-PTSD) symptoms, with several episodes consisting of my whole body shaking uncontrollably, a racing heart, freezing cold arms and legs as blood rushed to my major organs, a static-filled mind, nausea, diarrhea, constipation, and even vomiting. Within a few years I had 24/7 chronic fatigue and constant fibromyalgia flare-ups that could last weeks. All of this had been part of my life before I got into that relationship, but it was taken up many notches through the way my nervous system responded to our dynamic and how I was being treated. By the time I started coming out of denial, I had already been to the hospital with a bleeding stomach and was at the lowest emotional, physical, and spiritual bottom of my life. And that's saying a lot. I'm still recovering.

However, it wasn't all bad. We shared a love of filmmaking and acting, traveled extensively, spent time exploring the beauty of the natural world, taught meditation retreats together, had kitchen dance parties, late-night laughing fits, and profound mystical experiences together. Our connection inspired one of the most creatively abundant times of my life. I wrote a book, made multiple films, acted on stage and screen, and built my trauma-resolution business. The curious and playful way he interacted with children and how they always seemed to adore him made my ovaries ache. There was something magical about him and I felt proud to walk into a room with him. We were a handsome couple. We had great sex, though in hindsight I see our sex life in a less positive light. I believe that we loved each other to the degree that we were each capable of, though my idea of love is very different today.

Looking back, I see that my desire for him to put a ring on it was primarily based on a trauma bond and my strong attraction to what was familiar. I was born to a dad who would always choose alcohol over me and a mother who couldn't give me the love I desperately needed due to her own psychological distress. I didn't feel safe or consistently chosen and loved. My dad would disappear into intoxication, and my mother would disappear into dissociation and rage. I didn't feel consistently seen or prioritized. From very early on I was chasing after people who simply couldn't meet my basic emotional needs.

We have a biological imperative to be attracted to our primary caregivers in early development to ensure our survival, safety, and nurturing—even when we aren't safe or nurtured. My limbic system, where lust, love, and bonding chemicals reside, was wired to be attracted to what I associated with being loved and cared for: neglect, abuse, and chronic unpredictable stress. I believe this is why my strongest sexual and romantic attractions were toward (and best sex was with) people who experienced addiction and narcissistic and borderline personality disorders. I didn't tend to last long in relationships in which I was nurtured because I didn't *feel the spark*. The spark being created by brain chemistry related to an adverse childhood. My limbic brain resonated with what was familiar, even when that was to the detriment of my happiness and well-being. If I was starting to lose interest in someone, their best bet was to become less available and less enamored of me. It worked like an aphrodisiac love spell.

My long-term partner's inability to proclaim his love and commitment to me through this age-old ritual of marriage felt like home to me. I had been trained early in life to look for any hint of getting my needs met and to run after it. Trying to get just a taste of the dopamine, oxytocin, and endorphins I so desperately needed. This played out in the relationship and my strong desire to be chosen, accepted, and loved in the ways that felt most meaningful to me by someone who couldn't do it. He dropped just enough breadcrumbs, perhaps unintentionally, to keep me in a chronic state of hope though. He would give me a day or two of enthusiastic affection and words of affirmation after particularly bad instances of mistreatment, but often only after I took the blame for how he had treated me and apologized. It was a painful and addictive cycle that, given my limbic conditioning, seemed normal and like what I deserved. I went round after round, believing that it would change, denying what a wiser part of me knew. I tried to leave once but was too sick at the time to find the strength to overcome the addiction I had to our dynamic.

People stay for all kinds of reasons. Unless you are in it, you can't know what it's like, and any judgment is misplaced and misguided in my opinion. Once I thought I stayed for love, but now I know I stayed because of limbic resonance, cognitive dissonance, and a small child inside me who thought that if I could make him treat me well, choose me, and love me, it would make up for what my parents could not give me.

During my time in the hospital, *one day I'll have a kid* turned into a biological clock ringing loudly. I guess being that ill really connected me to my mortality and the drive to live and create more life. The other reason *baby* started flashing like a neon sign in my mind was that my partner showed up for me in a way that felt familial. His care seemed like that of a husband and the future father of my children. Not long after being discharged I became far more vocal about my desires, both to get married and to get knocked up. I was about to turn thirty-seven and we had been together for seven years. It was time, as far as I was concerned. The shifting goalposts and breadcrumbs continued, but now I was pushing back, and soon we became that couple who fought over marriage and kids, while our once spectacular sex life disintegrated.

I can only imagine that he struggled too. That perpetual state of indecision must have been painful for him. I'm not sure what level of self-awareness he had about the way he treated me, but even with what I would call an empathy deficit, it couldn't have felt good to see me crumple so often. Of course, my patience waned over the years, and I carried a low-level resentment in my eyes, my tone, my touch.

I tried my best to show up with love and kindness, even while feeling rejected and neglected, but I didn't always succeed. Our home became a dark place to reside. While I had some gargantuan chunks of anger about the way I was treated to work through, I can also have compassion for the suffering he must have been experiencing too.

I'm not proud of all my actions in that relationship. For example, because there had been some betrayals and fractures in trust, I turned to snooping occasionally. I looked at text and social media messages, which is absolutely a betrayal of trust and just not cool. When I did find what I was looking for, I didn't tell him that that I had discovered a dishonesty. I just pushed my feelings down, letting my resentment fester and my mistrust grow. I stopped doing that, and eventually, after we split, came clean and made amends, but by then the damage had been done. I certainly played my part in the dysfunction, and I am more than willing to claim the blame I own.

Interestingly, snooping was something that I did with both of my parents. I would look through their private drawers and shoeboxes in closets. I once found a pile of books my dad had about changing your identity and disappearing forever. At that time, he would often say that he was going to leave and never come back when he felt that me and my sisters were misbehaving. In my mother's bedroom I found a baby book with my name on it. What she had written about her challenges in caring for me as an infant, and her intrusive thoughts about me, were disturbing and heartbreaking. I suppose snooping was just another aspect of how I replayed parental patterns in my relationship.

I'm incredibly grateful that we never got married or had a child together. The person I am today can't fathom being in that relationship. When I left, it felt like I was running for my life. It had become undeniably clear one evening at a dinner party with two other couples who were obviously in much happier and healthier relationships than we were. The decision came all at once, but it wasn't sudden. I had asked again and again for what I wanted and needed, and again and again it was not available. I found us multiple couples therapists over the years, but we never made any progress. Often the focus would be shifted to me and my trauma rather than the real issues at hand. Not all couples therapists are trained to see triangulation and covert abuse. I stayed as long as I possibly could, holding out hope that a miracle would occur. I feel confident that I did everything I could. I also worked diligently, throughout those years, to heal the parts of me that associated love with neglect and abuse. I did psycho-spiritual brain surgery on myself. I revised my limbic brain's attraction and addiction to abusive relationships and people who were unable to choose me. This was a slow process, so slow that by the time I was ready to move on, the chances of conceiving without interventions had most likely moved on too. I spent my entire thirties in that relationship.

I'm not much for regrets. I can't change the past, and ruminating over it only makes things worse by pulling me out of the present and the choices I'll make that shape the future. I also love being me, and me is created by everything that came before. Plus regret is made of just thoughts and emotions, which are transient and impermanent phenomena, not the capital-T truth. I don't regret the years spent longing for something with someone who couldn't give it to me. I don't regret letting my childbearing years bleed out. But that doesn't mean I don't grieve the loss.

Yes, there are all kinds of options these days and it might be possible, but at what cost? Being a middle-aged single parent with a bunch of chronic conditions doesn't sound all that great to me. I also find it highly unlikely that in the very few years remaining to take advantage of the science of fertility I'll meet someone and take that plunge. Does this mean I don't really want a child? I don't think so. I just know how hard life can be sometimes taking care of my own inner child. Unless my bank account balance is miraculously a couple zeros higher in the next few years, even adoption won't be a viable option (I have some serious misgivings about the adoption industry anyway). If I put all my eggs in the baby basket, pun intended, I could find a way to be a parent, so I guess technically that makes me childless by choice. Though it doesn't always feel that way since I didn't choose my childhood or my chronic conditions, both of which impacted where I am now.

Something I have said to my clients, and that my therapists and coaches have needed to remind me of, is that trauma and chronic illness (and mental health struggles and undiagnosed neurodivergence) can change the traditional timeline of life. My limbic resonance with partners who were unable to treat me well, and my own avoidant behaviors with partners who could, found me in my forties before I had healed enough to leave that last relationship and consider the question of *what next*. Meanwhile many of my peers have a few kids and have already been married and divorced. Not that most of them don't have their own trauma and chronic conditions that have changed the trajectory of their lives. Perhaps some of them would be happily unmarried, with no kids by choice, if they had been untouched by the imprint of trauma or chronic conditions. I can't know for sure that I would have chosen children and marriage if I'd had an idyllic childhood and perfect health.

As I've reflected on this choice, or lack thereof, to be childless, I encountered a deep and surprising layer of grief about an abortion I had in 2000. When I got pregnant, I didn't even consider staying pregnant. I already had an appointment to start the termination process by the time I told my much, much older boyfriend that the pull-out method had failed us. I remember him looking stunned, but he didn't argue. I was so early in my pregnancy that I couldn't immediately get the procedure and had to wait longer than the state-mandated twenty-four hours. I remember one friend apologetically telling me that I was glowing during that time. I shut her down and changed the subject. I was intent on not getting attached to the clump of cells that were creating a fluttering feeling in my uterus. Interestingly, I stopped drinking and smoking for the weeks that I was pregnant. It was automatic.

I didn't consciously decide to pause my addictions, and I don't recall it being a challenge.

The day of my abortion, I allowed myself two minutes to cry. I buried my face in the futon couch in the living room of the apartment I shared with my much, much older boyfriend and sobbed. I heard myself say in a tearful whisper-scream, *I want to keep my baby, I want to keep my baby.* Then I got up, wiped off my face, and went down to the street to get in the car my much, much older boyfriend had idling in a loading zone. I opted for full anesthesia. I didn't want to remember a thing.

If I had made the choice to stay pregnant when I was twenty, I'd likely have an adult child now. I would have gone through the whole pregnancy and birth process, seen that baby turn into a kid, and that kid turn into a teen, and that teen turn into a young adult. I'd know the love and terror of parenthood. A part of me wishes I had not had the abortion.

It's been confusing to process that grief while pregnant people in the US are being stripped of their right to choose. When my health has allowed it, I've been protesting this human rights violation in the streets. I am unshakably pro-choice, pro–family planning, and pro–reproductive freedom. I believe that abortion is healthcare and I have held this belief since I was a child.

Once Trump was elected, I knew that *Roe v. Wade* would soon be overturned. It was only hanging on by a thread, and the religious right has had a death grip on the Republican party since Reagan. It was no surprise to me when the decision was leaked or when the ruling was announced. It's also been no surprise to see all the anti-trans legislation, book banning, and even the insurrection. Just like the tracks were laid for me to choose people who couldn't choose me, the tracks of fascism in the US were laid long ago. But I digress. Complicated feelings aside, it's been a strange time to second-guess the choice I made for my body over two decades ago.

But as I said, regret isn't really my jam. The truth is, I would have been a terrible, awful, no-good parent back then. I know this because I now know how much work it takes to resolve trauma and learn to live well with chronic conditions. It's taken me years, and incredible effort, to be where I am today. Back then I hadn't even begun to meaningfully address the symptoms of C-PTSD. Other than my brief and unexplainable stint of sobriety while I was pregnant, I was still in the jaws of addictive behaviors with drugs and alcohol. I hadn't yet realized that I was an extension of narcissism, which meant I hadn't yet learned to apologize and not to gaslight or love bomb. I didn't know how to work with my nervous system to remain in my window of tolerance during emotional challenges. I was years away from knowing how to take care of my body or manage my illnesses and pain. All that unexamined, unhealed, and unrecovered material would have infused my parenting. And it's not like I had parents, or any adults in my life, who could do any better than me.

I'd like to think I would have done a slightly better job than my parents did. Would I have physically or verbally abused my child? I hope not. Would I have been emotionally abusive and neglectful? It's very possible. Would I have taken my child into bars with me or driven with them in the car after a few drinks? Sadly, I probably would have. I wouldn't have been the worst parent on earth, not by a long shot, but I'm pretty sure that my child would now be dealing with the consequences of my poor parenting. They would have to go on to revise their own limbic systems if they wanted to have healthy functional relationships. Though I'm fairly confident that no matter how badly I fucked up as a parent, I would have loved that kid to the moon and back. Just as I don't regret having an abortion, I doubt that I would have ultimately regretted making the choice to stay pregnant.

As it is, I was only pregnant that once. For the years following that Dilaudid-drenched hospital stay, I wanted very badly to be pregnant again, but this time for the duration. If I was not in the habit of self-compassion and didn't know everything I know about the effects of trauma, I might blame myself for staying in that relationship. The truth is, I did the very best I could with the tools and capacity I had at that time. If I had been further along in my healing sooner, I would have left sooner. It's as simple as that.

The years of many types of trauma resolution, spiritual practice, and all the training I've had to be able to effectively and skillfully support my clients has changed my brain. It has changed what is acceptable for me in relationships of all kinds, including my romantic and sexual connections. I'd much rather hang out with my dog at home than with someone who isn't a match. I no longer get wet when someone who is visibly emotionally unavailable walks into the room. Inconsistency and fear of commitment bore rather than excite me. I can smell gaslighting from a mile away and I see right through love bombing. I've stopped falling for drugstore cowboys and daily drinkers. I don't date people who aren't enthusiastic about me and bubbling over to tell me so. Breadcrumbs does not a meal make, and dishonesty is a hard pass for me.

I spent so much time begging to be chosen, not realizing that I was the one who needed to do the choosing. Today I choose me. I choose me fiercely and with no hesitation. I deserve love, safety, and nurturing, so I give it to myself, to the best of my ability, every single day. I don't have a child, but I have myself. I can give myself the same love I would have given a child.

I am not a perfect parent to myself. Perfect parents don't exist. But I do a pretty good job a lot of the time. I feed myself nutritious food, drink plenty of water, put fresh sheets on my bed, take myself out to do fun things, set love-filled boundaries for myself, surround myself with safe and loving people. I learn, I rest, I prioritize well-being and thriving in all areas of my life. I don't do all these things without struggle 100 percent of the time. Sometimes basic self-care doesn't feel basic at all. I do my best, and when I can do better, I do better.

It doesn't look like I'll ever have a child, but I have two nephews and a niece who I love in a way that I think might be close to parental love. I am blessed to help my single-parent sister teach them that they are worthy of love and nurturing. I get the honor of being a consistent, safe, and trusted adult in their lives. I know firsthand how important that is. I also have a tiny, scruffy dog. I love him so much that I sometimes get dizzy and a little nauseous from the flood of love chemical he inspires in my brain. As my service dog, he takes care of me too. He is nine, and I have friends who are already preparing for when he dies. Dogs should really live a lot longer if you ask me. Along with those much-loved beings, I have clients who I offer a safe and supportive space to heal and learn in. This is quite different from a relationship with a child, as it should be of course. Still, it allows me an opportunity to express a nurturing side of myself and help others grow and thrive.

If I'm lucky I still have half a life left ahead of me. I may have missed some milestones, but I've also gained resilience and grit along the way. I know who I am and what matters to me, and I will never again bypass my truth for potential or hope. Limbic resonance, that primal and intricate dance of emotional connection, now revised, is no longer a tangle of scars and longing from the past. I've been reborn to myself: fresh, cherished, chosen.

The Migraine Years

The first time I prayed for death, I had a migraine. If you know migraines, you know them. There is something astonishing about this particular pain. It is truly awesome, as in the awesome power of the atom bomb. You cannot help but be bowled over by its breathtaking power. A migraine demands your submission and is enough to make you pray for deliverance through whatever means necessary, including a permanent vacation from this mortal coil.

The arrival of my migraines, first when I was a child, then in my late teens, and finally in my thirties, was not arbitrary; not in the least. My migraines held meaning, messengers of the sorrow and longing I could not express and the helplessness I could not escape.

That first time I felt the shock of pain inside my head and blinding shards of light attacking my retinas, I was seven or eight. My mother, who tirelessly worked multiple jobs to make ends meet, would often take me and my sisters with her to work. On this evening, I remember a chill in the air as we entered the building where she would attempt to sell toys and games, from a multilevel marketing company, to stay-at-home mothers. They wore pantyhose, had long shiny lacquered nails, sipped Diet Pepsis, and took small nibbles of buttery crackers with soft cheese. My mother, who hated pantyhose, wore pants, and had bare nails, which she had bit down to nubs. The drinks and snacks weren't for us.

I was to sit and watch the demonstration, a toy or two to occupy me. My sisters weren't with us this time, and that may have made me happy to have this special time with my mother. There were no other children, which couldn't have made much sense to me. I must have looked around and thought, *Why so many fun things for kids to play with and no kids in sight?* Out of nowhere, searing light sliced across my vision, partially blinding me. A dizzy and nauseous feeling set in.

I knew not to interrupt my mother's demonstration, not with all these fancy ladies here. But soon I had no choice but to tug at her sleeve. My head had begun to throb and ache, but it was so much worse than the headaches I often had. I had never felt anything quite like it and I was afraid. The fluorescent lights were a medieval torture device. Every crunch of a cracker or shuffle of paper was a crowbar to my brain.

I don't remember how my mother excused herself. I don't remember if I threw up like I sometimes do when a migraine hits. I don't remember getting back into the car, but I do recall the short moment of relief in darkness and cool air of night. I remember my mother going back inside. She had to finish the job, or at least pack up the toys. How long was she gone? Fifteen minutes, two hours, a year? Time no longer made sense. Nothing made sense. Reality was a confusing cubist painting, everything I knew jumbled. One thing was clear, I desperately needed the pain to stop. I begged, small hands squeezed into fists, alone in that dark, cold car. I begged to be released from the unfamiliar suffering. I begged to disappear so that I could no longer feel anything.

The migraines continued that year. The most memorable was on the Fourth of July. We had moved into my mother's boyfriend's house, and our blended family went to the neighbors to watch their backyard fireworks show. I was alone at home in bed, my open windows facing the festivities. The booming explosions and flashing lights flew into my room and ricocheted between the walls. The pain was unfathomable. I remember wishing that someone would smash my head open with a hammer. I imagined my scalp splitting, my skull cracking, and pink brain becoming mushy like oatmeal. It seemed a better option than what I was experiencing. That hammer wouldn't just cure the migraines, perhaps it could save me from the other turns life had been taking lately.

It's hard to believe that the adults in my life didn't recognize the significance of the timing of this new malady of mine. My migraines began a few years after my parents split up. My mother was fed up with my father's drinking and in love with a man with a ponytail, a big house, and two sons. The exhaustion of living with an alcoholic, albeit a sweet and silly alcoholic, and the new relationship energy pumping through her body were enough to make her pack up and move out, my sisters and me in tow. We left behind the house our parents had been so proud to buy. The house they had told us was our home. My father fell into a darker phase of addiction, adding unprescribed Xanax and Percocet to his daily self-medication regimen. Child support was almost nonexistent, though my parents were in and out of court over it, generally bringing us along for the show. The small basement apartment my mother could afford had cockroaches, cement floors, and a landlord upstairs who beat her son until his screams turned to eerie silence. In a heartbreaking turn of events years later, that abused child went on to beat his own child to death. We lived beneath the consequences of generational trauma that I can't bear to even begin to fathom. Still, at only six years old, I did my best to make it feel like my home.

At Christmastime I was at the apartment alone and saw the violent landlord lugging a big live tree up the driveway and into her house above us. My mother had said we wouldn't be getting a tree that year, too expensive. With my nose against the icy glass window, I watched as a few small branches fell to the asphalt. As soon as I heard her door close, I scampered outside and gathered the green piney branches. I found the Scotch tape in the kitchen drawer and, careful not to use too much, I fixed the bits of tree to the wall. Then I made decorations and fake presents out of colored construction paper and markers. I surprised my mother and sisters with our *Christmas Tree* when they came home. Did it delight my mother or break her heart? Was she too tired to even care? I don't know. But I was making the best of a bad situation by inviting some holiday spirit to visit.

My mother's boyfriend would also come to visit. I didn't trust him, and I didn't understand why he was there, this guy who my parents had invited along on a camping trip earlier that year. This guy had blown out his knee swimming in the ocean and my father had brought him safely back to shore. Later, my father screamed his name at my mother: *I never should have saved him. I should have let him drown.* What was this guy doing sitting on our thinly carpeted concrete floor? Why was he trying to get me to like him? I remember spilling a drink and he quickly cleaned it up, saying, *We just won't let your mom know about that.* Why was this guy telling me to lie to my mother?

Our second apartment was so much better. It was on the second floor, and I had my own room. My sisters, only five and two, slept in the other bedroom with my mother. Right across the street was a little park with a mossy-banked stream and lots of places to pretend to be a royal fairy or Luke Skywalker. Sun streamed in the windows. My mother smiled more. The best part was that my father came to visit sometimes too, not just the new boyfriend. At Christmastime we had a tree and my mother left oats sprinkled on the wall-to-wall carpet for us to find the next morning. Santa had come and some of the food for his reindeer had spilled, she told us. I already knew that there was no Santa, but she didn't know that and I liked pretending that I didn't either. It was a mostly sweet time in that apartment, a reprieve from the chaos that had come with my parents splitting up.

Then something changed. My father stopped coming and the boy-friend came more often. My father, devastated and furious, formed an alliance with the downstairs neighbor to make my mother's life miserable, and our neighbor, sick of the sound of children running around above her, was happy to oblige. She blew cigarette smoke under our door, made rude comments, watched my mother's every move and reported back to my father, and once even called the cops. My mother had left me in charge of my sisters and went to the store up the street. The spying neighbor saw her leave and made a call citing young children left alone at night. While of course a seven-year-old has no business babysitting two small children, matters weren't improved by a knock on the door from two officers. My mother had returned home in the nick of time and was there to answer the door, assuring them all was well.

All was not well. She was pregnant with her boyfriend's child, being terrorized by a chain-smoking cop-calling neighbor, and trying to support three young children—and to add insult to injury, her car was nearly totaled in front of the apartment building in a hit-and-run. Her smiles were not as easy to come by anymore. But she had an out. Her boyfriend had been asking her to move into his big house, making one big *Brady Bunch*–style family for a while now.

My mother had to bribe me to go to there to visit. I once wedged myself between a piece of furniture and the wall, refusing to come out and get in the car to go to his house. I finally gave in when she offered me a bulk pack of Reese's Peanut Butter Cups, all to myself. I guess integrity goes right out the window for such a large quantity of candy at that age. I didn't like going to his house. I didn't like the dusty, thick smell. I didn't like the fleas on the area rugs that bit my legs and ankles. I didn't like the edge that had started to creep into his voice when he didn't approve of something one of my sisters or I did. I didn't like the way my mother's voice sounded pretend, but not like a royal fairy or Luke Skywalker. She sounded like who he wanted her to be, even to my young ears. I didn't like when we slept over and she would sneak off to his bedroom before I fell asleep. She didn't tell me her plans until the day we moved. She knew I wouldn't be happy about it. I knew it wasn't a place to call home.

I came home from a weekend trip to my father's to see my things being loaded into the back of the boyfriend's brown pickup truck. In went my rainbow suitcase. In went my bed frame with the Smurf stickers on the headboard. In went my green teddy bear and the rest of my stuffed animals stuffed in a white plastic bag. Smiles spread on adults' mouths like melted candy. I tucked my silent gasp into my sinking heart and willed myself not to cry, ashamed that I had been surprised.

All of this was the unhappy seed planted inside my head that later blossomed into blinding pain, suddenly and without mercy, forcing me to the darkness of the car, while my mother sold toys to other mothers inside a fluorescent-lit room. The rainbow suitcase and teddy bear eyes looking out of a white plastic bag turned to screaming fights; to thumbprint bruises blossoming on small pale arms; to a house full of eggshells. My mother's eyes went vacant for days; or worse she closed her bedroom door, her sobbing seeping down the staircase. Her anger became more vicious and made its way to my body more often than before. *You're an asshole* spat from her lips. The migraines, I know now, were an obvious case of cause and effect. I was affected, but less and less surprised.

My mother tried homeopathy to cure me. The little sugar pills did nothing but leave a much-needed sweetness under my tongue. Eventually there was talk of taking me to Children's Hospital in the city. I hoped they would take me because a hospital just for children sounded like a wonderful place to be. When the migraines disappeared as quickly as they had arrived, I was relieved but also disappointed. The migraines expressed a constant pain I felt but had no words for. Having a name for it made it easier to endure somehow. My pain would, of course, find new ways to express.

The memory of the migraines remained, unmoving. Animal-level pain leaves dark stains. Chronic tension headaches replaced the migraines and continue to this day. I didn't have another migraine until the day my father called me in 2005 to tell me he had cancer, too drunk to speak, crying too hard to try. Angry and afraid, I screamed at him. He had done this to himself.

I hung up, heavy with guilt, devastated, seeing stars that turned to lightning, that turned to old stains of pain becoming fresh and wet. I knew what was coming this time. I'd never forgotten the way a migraine announced itself.

New to LA and more or less alone, I only had my new girlfriend to turn to for soothing and support. My new girlfriend and *her* house full of eggshells. My new girlfriend who called me an asshole and told me to move back to Pennsylvania when I misstepped and one of the eggshells crunched. I went to her, and she tried her best to comfort me, uncomfortable as she was with another person's pain. I tried my best to keep myself small and still, not to let her know how much agony I was in, even though fireworks were going off inside my skull. I sat next to her and pretended to watch TV with her housemates, closing my eyes when she wasn't looking, longing for a cool dark room, or at least a car. The fear of her punishment was almost worse than the pain.

By this time I had done enough therapy and read enough self-help books to assume that the cause of this migraine was the news I had received from my father. I hadn't healed enough to know that the effects of this abusive relationship were maybe the more prominent cause. Finding out your father has cancer with a supportive and loving partner is already migraine worthy on its own, but adding this circumstance was another beast altogether. I wrestled it until it calmed, its snarls softening.

Then five or six years later, a few years after my father died, the migraines came back full force. They became chronic. I saw neurologists, took preventative medications, and found myself in urgent care more than once for pain that lasted over forty-eight hours. They had returned just a month or two into a new relationship. I didn't see the cause and effect. I was in love, and it felt like home to be in his arms. It felt like home to see his eyes go vacant and look right through me. It felt like home to have carpets of eggshells beneath my feet again. It felt like the home that I hid behind chairs to avoid. It felt like a home of shameful surprises and seeds of pain.

For several years I did not recognize the meaning of these migraines. I didn't yet know them as messengers, though they spoke loudly of sorrow and longing. I had learned to remain helpless, with no taste for escape, and this blinded me more than the searing pain coursing through my head. Dark rooms, prayers for release, narcotics. Useless. I made the home I knew how to make, but now I was too tired to gather pine tree branches and Scotch tape.

I look back now and marvel at how oblivious I was. No different from the adults who couldn't put together the simple puzzle of my migraines. Who couldn't see that their inability to heal themselves was harming me. I have compassion for them now. When my inability to heal, and to change my definition of home and love, was hurting me, I was already older than they had been when my migraines began. How could they have known? And how could I have known?

When I was eight, my mother's boyfriend was the villain, the reason for my mother's deep grief and unpredictable rage. The cause of my pain. Now, though they never married, he is her lifelong partner, and I call him my stepfather. I see now how they both played their parts in what happened inside the walls of that house. They both sprinkled eggshells on the hardwood floors and flea-filled area rugs. I see how they both wanted to be better for us kids. I learned later that they had gone to parenting classes to learn how to manage stress and anger. I feel a sad tenderness imagining them in a florescent-lit room in the late eighties, listening to a woman in pantyhose talk about taking three deep breaths when mad instead of slapping your child. I'm not close with my stepfather or my mother, but I understand now that there are no villains, only flawed humans trying to put together the puzzles of their lives with as much grace as they could, me included.

Those last migraine years eventually sputtered out. The messengers lost steam and slowed down when I introduced them to cannabis, but many new messengers took their place, until my entire body was messages made of pain. I started to listen, with great resistance at first, but soon I could hear the sorrow and the longing. There was a great sadness about what I had been taught to call home being expressed by my pain. I had settled for so much less than what I needed or deserved because I didn't know that what I came from was far from nurturing. I longed for a true home, filled with love, peace, and soft places to rest my aching head and heart. I needed safety and consistency. When I could finally read the messages my body was sending me, there was no option to return to sender. I had to surrender. I could no longer tuck silent gasps into my sinking heart. I couldn't turn off the tears if they needed to flow. When my name was traded for words meant to hurt, or someone's unkindness or a lack of empathy surprised me, I no longer shrunk in shame. The helplessness was seen for what it was: learned, which meant it could be unlearned.

This unlearning showed me how to build a new kind of home inside myself. A home that can't be taken away from me or filled with eggshells and violent words. I choose who to allow in and who to keep out. Shaming and withholding do not mingle with love. In my home, I don't have to hide my pain or shrink to be deemed acceptable. I am not bribed by sweetness, instead it is freely given without expectation. Soft sunshine and sounds of water over smooth stones stream in. Rainbow light travels across the walls. Here I know that love doesn't need to feel like a head full of hammers and fireworks. As an adult I've learned that adverse childhood experiences have been shown to cause frequent headaches in adults.[1] I've learned how to address this consequence of my history with love.

My migraine years were signals that I didn't feel safe, loved, and seen. That inhumane pain was a message of human need. When I was small and before I understood the reason for the pain, I had no way to read the writing and reply. Some days in giving myself what I need, I don't sleep enough or drink enough water or get enough calories or ask for enough help and care from those who would gladly offer it. A black-and-white rerun of deprivation. I forget that the way I was once treated is not how I must treat myself. Some days I forget that my home is mine, to be filled with love that can heal, not hurt. At these times a messenger arrives carrying a scroll of pain, but now I can read it and I understand how to reply.

When I hear the knock of a migraine messenger at my door, the sound is familiar, now crystal clear in its meaning. When my head starts to ache, I know the message written in the pain. It tells me that I am safe, loved, and seen, and unconditionally deserving of the sweetness of home. That I am not required to wear a crown of pain to belong, and that the care I need is available to me.

If I listen to the message early enough, a meal, a glass of water, or a forgotten daily medication might be all that is needed. If I wait, forgetting that I don't need to deprive myself of basic care, there will be a painful reminder that can last for hours until I am able to soothe it with cannabis and sleep. Of course, the reason for these messages isn't always as simple as a missed meal, medication, or dehydration. Often my response must be one of self-compassionate action. I may need to take a break from the news, reach out to a trusted friend, consciously grieve, cut a few things from an overscheduled week, find ways to express my creativity if it's been pushed aside for other things, or just get under the blankets and watch good TV. Occasionally a headache will appear to let me know that something, or someone, must be let go of. I don't always want to listen to those messages, but I know the cost of holding on to what is not aligned for my highest good. Sometimes a head full of pain is simply marking a time of change and transformation. These messages are growing pains, and on the other side I feel even more at home.

The message is loud and clear, and I am listening.

The message is trustworthy, and so I trust it.

Spoons

I am low on spoons, and I don't mean the sort of spoons you eat soup with. Speaking of soup, I do need some chicken soup, because I have an unhappy stomach. A simple chicken soup is pretty much all I can eat when I feel sick. But I haven't made any lately, so there is not a stockpile of broth-filled mason jars in my freezer. I haven't made any lately because I let the chicken I was going to use go bad in the fridge (I feel guilty about this useless death). And the chicken before that was used for some internet recipe that was too flavorful for me and had soy, which I don't even eat. I gave it to my neighbor.

So now I'd have to go out and buy chicken, and then prepare the soup, and then jar the soup. I'd also have to work through the disgust I have with raw chicken. Because I have a few things that I need to do later today, I do not have the spoons to get in the car, shop, drive home, and then prepare, and jar the broth. I really don't have the spoons to digest the disgust, especially since I'm nauseous already. I'm considering having a jar of chicken soup from Erewhon Market (an absolutely ridiculously expensive grocery store that gets made fun of on social media for its $20 smoothies) delivered, but each time I try to complete the order I think of my credit card bills and I don't do it. It's taking a lot of self-compassion to keep from scolding myself for spending all my spoons and all my money and being in this position at the present.

Oh, sweet spoonie. Some days are just like this. It will get better. It's ohhhh-kay, baby.

The Spoon Theory was created by Christine Miserandino in 2003.[1] A friend wanted to know what it was like to live with lupus, and Miserandino used spoons as a metaphor for having a limited amount of energy each day. Each activity, including self-care, work, and play, costs a certain number of spoons. If you run out, even brushing your teeth can be impossible. A person living without a chronic condition doesn't need to consider how many spoons they have, or how many spoons a specific activity will cost. Spoonies do.

I am a spoonie. I am sometimes a bad spoonie (I say *bad* with kindness and because it sounds funny to me, *bad spoonie*) because even after all these years, I forget that I don't have endless spoons. I forget that I don't necessarily have the same number of spoons every day. I forget to save contingency spoons. I forget that something as simple as a change in weather, a strong smell that hits wrong, or an unexpected bright light can deplete all my spoons in one fell swoop. I forget what happens when I try to reuse a dirty spoon or just go spoonless (it's not pretty). I forget that most people don't even know what the hell I'm talking about when I say *I'm out of spoons today.* (*You're what?*) I forget that I always need chicken soup in the freezer.

You better believe that I remember right quick when my spoons are dwindling. Let's do some spoon math. Start with the idea that my average number of spoons is fourteen. It can be a bit higher on a great day and a lot lower on a rotten day. Today I woke up below my average. Why? Because I was low on spoons yesterday too, and so I got distracted by a TV show and went to bed too late. Overspending spoons is a cumulative slippery slope, which can end in a big flare-up. I had twelve spoons this morning. Here's how I've been spending them so far:

+ Woke up and saw immediately that my internet was out. The stress of that cost me a spoon. If it were a client day, it would have cost me quite a few more as I'd need to reschedule folks, and that is stressful. For me, stress is equal to spoons spent.

✦ I also woke up to a very unhappy stomach. My gastrointestinal distress is at an eight. This is part of the reason my spoons are low and it cost a spoon to manage.

✦ Making breakfast (which I could barely eat due to the unhappy stomach), brushing my teeth, morning skincare, taking my meds, and walking my dog cost another spoon.

✦ I had therapy (a phone session, because no internet). I love therapy. Because I hold space for my clients it's important that space is also held for me. Plus I've always loved being attended to and cared for in the way I am with a good therapist or coach. Nonetheless, it cost me a spoon to have the session, as we tapped into some deep grief.

✦ Then I had some unexpected work to do for an acting class I teach, a client needed some text support, and a friend needed some text support, and I had a few long emails to reply to. (Inboxes are the bane of my existence. In fact, back in the late '90s–early 2000s I refused to use email, much to my colleagues' dismay. I can't get away with that today.) Some of this involved stress. This all cost me two spoons. That's six spoons before noon. With these six remaining spoons, I must be *very* intentional. I must be *very* slow. I must ooze with self-care, love, and compassion. I'd like to go to a church event tonight, which could potentially *give* me a spoon or two. Spiritual practice, massages, *some* social interactions, and activities of that nature can give me a fresh spoon, *if* I'm not too depleted. This is why I will prioritize going to church tonight. But I need to make it to this evening with at least three spoons to drive there, socialize, drive home, and do my bedtime self-care. That means I have three spoons for the entire afternoon. This is where the power of *No* comes in.

The power of no is something that all spoonies must learn to wield (and learn again, and again). Once upon a time I was unable to say no, which meant I was always depleted and often resentful. A huge reason for my careless yeses was that I had a combo of FOMO (fear of missing out) and a case of the capitalist blues. I said yes to social interactions and low-paid and unpaid creative work because I was afraid that I'd miss out on something really fun or an opportunity that would lead to paid creative work.

I would find myself booked for multiple coffees, hikes, and the like in a single week. Running all over town and not actually having the spoons to engage in so much social activity, which often required exhausting masking of pain and neurodivergence, led to low-quality interactions with people who I would have liked to give my full presence to. So I ended up missing out anyway. Same with acting. I took *jobs* that couldn't even afford to feed me well, let alone pay me. Because I wasn't well-resourced, some of those performances were not my best, which didn't help my acting career all that much.

Feeling compelled to say yes to work because I live in a system that requires you work for a living (*life is for those who can pay for it*) kept me in a cycle of burnout from the time I was a teenager until I was in my thirties. The epitome of this was when I was both a nanny and a dog walker. I was wrangling three dogs in the rain and pushing a stroller through soggy grass, while nearly doubled over in pain from a UTI. When I ran theater companies in Philadelphia, I worked seven days a week and the theater was three blocks from where I lived. I once told my girlfriend that it was unreasonable of her to ask me to take off for holidays or birthdays. During that time, I was also acting, running a monthly queer party, and cleaning the floors of a data storage farm in the wee hours. Back then I had to work multiple jobs, but there were ways I could have adjusted my relationship with work, had I the ability to say no.

A propensity for people-pleasing also left me feeling choiceless and drained. I used to say yes anytime someone asked to *pick my brain* (ouch). I said yes to spending time with people I didn't feel aligned with but wanted to be friends. I said yes to people who used me as a free therapist. I said yes to therapists who weren't helping me, not wanting to hurt their feelings. I said yes to sex with people I wasn't attracted to, to family requests that weren't my responsibility, and yes to feeding cats and housesitting for casual acquaintances who were traveling, when I was already neglecting my own cats and house. I said yes to a lot of things I didn't want to do, or even care much about, all in the name of pleasing others. And let's be honest, that kind of pleasing isn't generous. It's steeped in resentment and it's dishonest.

A big gift of being a spoonie is that eventually I had no option but to start saying no. I was out of spoons. It was time to harness the power of no. It was painfully challenging at first, and I fell off the no wagon time and time again. My body kept giving me clear messages that I needed to let go of FOMO, my fear- and scarcity-based decision making, and people-pleasing. The messages got louder and louder, and the consequences of not listening got greater and greater. Eventually I understood that *No.* is a complete sentence and that I could say it while still socializing, creating art, making money, and being a kind and generous person. Of course, when you stop people- pleasing, some people stop being pleased. But the folks who actually care about your well-being and have been rooting for you to own your no will be quite pleased. Al-Anon, the 12-step program for loved ones of alcoholics, and books like Melody Beattie's *Codependent No More* are great supports for recovering from people-pleasing.

For the most part I stopped saying yes to anything that I was doing out of fear, didn't want to do, or didn't care about. Of course, I still must make money, but the power of no has made room for work that I am passionate about and that pays me handsomely. In more recent years I've had to learn to say no to things that I really want to do. That has also been a process, one that I am still in. It can be quite painful to walk away from something that lights me up inside, but the things I say no to shape the life I have, and life is good. I recognize I am very privileged to be in this position. While I've worked hard in a multitude of ways to arrive here, the color of my skin, among other factors, has afforded me opportunities and resources that I would not have otherwise had.

Spoonies who experience the direct effects of systemic racism likely spend more spoons than me every time they drive their car, because of how Black and brown bodies are treated by the police. That stress can be expensive in spoons. Each microaggression a spoonie of color is exposed to might cost a spoon or two. The embodied generational trauma that comes from being Black in America might make a spoonie more susceptible to being chronically low on spoons. I have no doubt that navigating much of the healthcare system costs more spoons for people who don't have the privilege of whiteness, and spoonies spend a lot of time in doctor's offices. It costs spoons to live in this world with Black or brown skin. I don't incur that cost.

I'm not sure that I would have recognized the power of no if I wasn't a spoonie. Between my conditioning from a traumatic childhood, the systems that harm that I exist inside of, and my neurodivergent tendency to spread myself in too many different directions, I may have gone on for some time feeling overwhelmed, resentful, and disconnected from the truth about what held value and joy for me. However, I am a spoonie. And this spoonie is going to say a whole bunch of no today, so that I can get my ass to church tonight.

+ I say no to a call with a friend who is having relationship issues. I schedule it for another day when I will be able to be a great pal.

+ I say no to listening to the voice notes from friends and family that have been piling up since yesterday. I will enjoy them and send better replies when I have the spoons.

+ I say no to any sort of strenuous exercise and instead do some gentle stretching.

+ I say no to shopping for chicken, but also say no to spending money I don't have, and choose to spend one spoon on making a very simple and very weird soup with heart of palm noodles, vegetable broth, carrots, and peas. Once I eat, I feel a lot better.

+ I say no to looking at my to-do list, and instead focus solely on the most important project that has a hard deadline. Because I get into an energetic and hyperfixated state, and I enjoy this project, I don't seem to lose any spoons.

- ✦ I say no to social media. A little doesn't have to cost spoons, but when I fall into the rabbit hole of ADHD TikTok and anti-capitalist Reddit, the Queen of Fatigue yells, "Off with their head!"

- ✦ I kindly say no to self-judgment. *Sweet spoonie, you are doing a great job.*

- ✦ I give myself the option to *not* go to church and play it by ear. This takes away any pressure to be ready at a particular time, or if I spend more spoons and need the last one for getting myself ready for bed. I make it to church, get filled with the Spirit, and gain a spoon. Hallelujah! This means I have an extra spoon to listen to my little sister's voice notes about a date she went on and reply with some unsolicited advice. Older siblings do that sometimes. This day could have gone very differently if I hadn't managed my spoons. I could have not only missed church and the voice note exchange with my sister, but by the time I went to bed I could have been in massive pain. Today was a spoonie victory.

Victories are measured day-to-day, not based on what made me feel victorious last week. Sometimes just getting out of bed is a win and sometimes international travel is a win. Becoming comfortable going with the flow is another big spoonie gift. Chronic illness can be a wild and unpredictable river. When we don't know what the next hour may bring (though who really does!), we are invited to embrace and accept the present moment. Some of the lowest periods of my physical and mental health have led to profound shifts into acceptance and presence. The capacity to have deeper compassion for others is also a perk of being in the spoonie club.

When you know the grief of lost dreams and opportunities, the agony of pain that never stops, and the experience of living in a world built for the able-bodied, you are more likely to remember this oft-quoted phrase: *Everyone you meet is fighting a battle you know nothing about. Be kind. Always.* Fellow spoonies are some of the kindest and most compassionate people I have ever met. The online and IRL spoonie communities are off the hook. We look out for each other, root for each other, cry, celebrate, and create with each other. We aren't afraid of seeing suffering or speaking up for unkindness and injustice.

I think that the years of being pummeled by pain and the unpredictability of chronic conditions have tenderized me and made me kinder and more attuned to others' suffering. I've also had the opportunity to know what it's like to be sick, experience mental health issues, and be neurodivergent in America. While there's much I can never know, oppression and prejudice that will never affect me, my lived experience helps me better understand the effects of harmful systemic systems and structures of this world. I know many spoonies who are activists, and not only for disability rights.

Spoonies aren't just people with chronic illness. The spoon theory works for those of us who are neurodivergent or experience anxiety, depression, the effects of C-PTSD, or any other mental health condition. A high-anxiety day might mean there are not enough spoons to deal with any tasks that could potentially create more anxiety. You might need to hunker down with a funny movie and some comfort food. When depression is a blanket made of concrete laid on your chest, you just might not have the spoons to *take a walk* or do any of the other things your well-meaning friends and family may suggest. Trying to do more than your depressed state will allow can deplete the few spoons you have. As good as cardio might be for creating happy chemicals, lying on the floor and doing a few slow and easy stretches might be what you need to conserve the spoons for a walk or a call with a loved one tomorrow.

For me, it's possible to gain spoons through regenerative activities and experiences. I find it helpful to have a list of potential spoon replenishers. That list is fluid, and what works one day may not work the next. A few of my favorites are: cuddling my dog; resting with sleep, music, or yoga nidra for an hour; a massage; certain types of meditation; time spent in nature; and, rarely, spending time with other people. All have the potential to replenish my spoons.

I try to be strategic about my days and plan to have spoons left at the end of the day to give my future self a nice start the next morning. I do a quick tidying up so that there's no clutter or dirty dishes. I get my stovetop espresso maker clean, if not packed and ready to go. I make myself some lemon water and prepare my morning medications and supplements. I take my dog out for one last pee so he will sleep longer the next day. Waking up with all of this prepared means I don't immediately lose spoons. The lack of clutter and dishes in the sink alone saves me stress that would cost me valuable spoonage.

I plan my days. I time-block. I'm not always the best at this, but when I do it, oh how well it works. Time blocking keeps me from wondering what I'm supposed to be doing, so I don't end up draining my energy multitasking and scrolling. I don't see more than four clients a day, and don't tend to do anything social on client days. I don't see clients any earlier than 10:30 a.m. Unless it's unavoidable, I don't schedule *anything* out of the house earlier than 11 a.m. I only drive if I must, and only stack two or three errands in one day if they are in the same area. I ask friends to visit me at my home or go to theirs instead of at a café, which involves a lot more stimuli. Still, I don't burden myself with an attachment to strict morning, afternoon, or evening routines. While I can totally understand the benefit of routine and structure, and implement that as much as possible, I'd rather be relaxed and joyful than force a *miracle morning* or hold tight to an idea of how my day *should* look. Rigid routines are laughable given the ever-changing nature of spoonie life.

Speaking of laughing, spoonies often have a delightfully dark sense of humor. I follow several social media accounts that post hilarious memes about the difficulties of dealing with doctors who don't listen, the side effects of medications, executive disfunction, autistic burnout, and living with chronic pain. We poke fun at ourselves, our aching bodies, our foggy brains, and at the well-meaning friends and family who say the least helpful things. We spoonies are not a glum lot. We laugh at things that make non-spoonies gasp loudly and say,

I'm so sorry, that must be so hard! When I can cackle with someone about our childhood traumas and how many meds we've tried for our migraines, I know I'm in good company.

The company I keep and the things I invest myself in are not arbitrary or accidental. When most things cost a spoon or two, I'm intentional with how I use my time and energy. This is yet another gift of being a spoonie. I know what holds meaning and purpose for me and how to prioritize based on that. For me, living with chronic conditions doesn't allow for mediocre connections. This makes me more discerning about the relationships I choose to nurture. That goes for friends, clients, colleagues, one-night stands, partners, and even family members. If we can't be authentic, vulnerable, and intimate (there are different versions of intimate of course), I can't fuck with you. I spend my spoons on people who want to see me and be seen by me.

My spoons are precious and so are the people and activities I spend them on. The fact that I have limited capacity for friends, dating, creative projects, and clients means that when I say yes to something, it's something I really want. For this reason, I am aware of what I mean to the spoonies in my life too. We are choosing each other, and that is something to be grateful for.

Yes, it sucks to be a spoonie, but that's only one shade of a many-hued existence. Being a spoonie comes with community, discernment, gratitude, open-mindedness, humor, compassion, intentionality, kindness, meaning, and purpose. Us spoonies don't take the small pleasures and micro wins for granted. We know how to live. We are willing to keep showing up, one day at a time, even when our good vein stops cooperating with the endless blood draws or a meltdown is looming. We love life even when it gives us the world's largest spoonful of lemons. Ain't nothing like some spoonie lemonade. Or chicken soup.

My Fucking Back Hurts

Red lipstick, black patent leather stilettos, sheer back-seamed stockings hooked to a garter belt, and nothing else. Back arched, abs tight, face relaxed, sex-eyes bright. The camera flashes again and again. The photographer doesn't know that I have taken every kind of painkiller I have: muscle relaxants, narcotics, cannabis-infused mints, topical ointments, mindfulness, dissociation. None of it can touch the pain. Consistent in my lower back, with sharp spikes every few minutes. One move the wrong way and I lose my breath. It turns my stomach. Am I going to pass out? My fucking back hurts.

Has my back ever not hurt? Not that I can recall. I had knots in my shoulders and in the muscles along my spine from the time I could say *it hurts*. Was that my first full sentence? Unlikely, but may as well have been. Over the years I got used to the pain and found ways to alleviate it. Massage, Epsom salt baths, meditation, medication, yoga. It became manageable.

I knew about back pain. I knew how to deal with back pain. At least I thought I did. That day on set modeling, I found out how naive I had been. I had never really known what true lower back pain was, but nearly naked and in front of a clicking camera, I found out.

There had been foreshadowing. A few weeks before, I walked a red carpet for a film I was in, went to the afterparty, and by the end of the evening was experiencing a *new* pain in my lower back. When you have chronic pain, a new symptom is like the inception of an anti-holiday. In anti-celebration we cry out, *What is this fresh hell?!* If the symptom becomes chronic, we can mark the day when it first began. This lower back pain subsided in less than a day, and I chalked it up to too many hours in high heels. I had already greatly limited my heel use because poor posture in a barre class had left me with the beginnings of bunions, and fuck that. But now and then seemed to be fine, and certainly for a film premiere. When the pain passed, I counted my blessings and moved on.

Then, much to my disappointment, came my brand-new anti-holiday. The shoot started out fine, but out of nowhere that pain I had felt at the premiere was back with a vengeance and growing. I started popping pills, trying to stay ahead of the pain. A big part of pain management with medication is taking it *before* the pain becomes overwhelming. I didn't come close to keeping up with that pain that day. It was at a ten before my pills even kicked in. I added the rest of my arsenal of anesthetizing agents, I needed to get through this shoot. No luck. I ended up foggy headed and droopy eyed, and still in just as much pain.

That was a turning point for me. I had been using narcotics daily for over a year, and up until then they had mostly worked. They allowed me to model, walk red carpets, date multiple people, work out, go on a book tour, fuck, make films, and be in the world even with my chronic conditions. At least that's the way I looked at it at the time. In hindsight, I'd add that the daily narcotic use also allowed me to push past what was safe or healthy for my body. They dulled my emotions and exacerbated my IBS symptoms. I was also worried that the opioid epidemic and the changes in the medical field would cut off my supply and I'd have to go off them cold turkey, which didn't sound like a good time.

As it was, I ended up going cold turkey of my own accord. As I was striking another painful pose on set, getting no relief from the medication, I thought, *What is the fucking point of narcotics if they can't make this pain stop?* As the pain continued for days after the modeling job, I didn't bother with the narcotics. When the pain was unrelenting after a trip to my physical therapist, and another few days, I headed to urgent care. After some imaging of my spine, I went to see a doctor to get the results.

He had a gaslighting-style bedside manner. The imaging showed that I had degenerative disc disease. When I told the doctor how terrible and debilitating the pain was, he responded that I only had a *little* degeneration, and that *it really shouldn't hurt that much.* I started to think he either hadn't read my chart or had but was a doctor who didn't take fibromyalgia seriously. For me, something that might not be noticeable at all for someone else could be incredibly painful due to the way my brain processes pain. I informed him that yes indeed it *did* hurt that much, to which he sighed and looked at the ceiling. He told me it really wasn't a big deal and many people had degenerative disc disease (one-third of people show signs by age forty[1]) and didn't experience pain at all. I gave up, having no interest in attempting to convince this man of my pain level. I did let him know that I had stopped using the narcotics, but that I needed a refill on my muscle relaxants.

You'd think that the fact that I wasn't asking for narcotics should have been a clue that I wasn't a drug-seeking client, but he made me ask several times for the drug I was regularly prescribed. When he suggested ibuprofen, it became obvious he hadn't read my chart, which clearly stated I could not take nonsteroidal anti-inflammatories because of the bleeding stomach I'd had a few years back. I wish I could say he was the only doctor who ever treated me that way, but I'd be telling a tall tale.

After finding out the reason my fucking back hurt so bad, I started getting physical therapy regularly, boxed up my heels, took a hiatus from modeling, and stopped exercising. Finally, the pain passed and I celebrated with a hard, fast, rough fuck. That's when the reality of my situation became crystal clear. I couldn't walk for days, and not in the good way. My back hurt worse than it had the day on set, or any day ever, save after a bad car accident years earlier. What may have hurt worse was the realization that I couldn't fuck like a porn star anymore, and that this back pain, added to all my other chronic issues, was going to stop my life as I knew it.

That led to a period when I was 80 percent homebound. This new symptom was the straw that broke the camel's back (and mine too). I saved my energy for work travel and clients and closed out my social life for the most part. I said no to all sorts of opportunities. I stopped dating anyone other than my partner who I lived with. I had very little sex. I stopped driving. Every time I would extend myself, even the smallest amount, my lower back pain would rise fast and furious, like a bat out of hell. It would take days to subside.

I started to try to get used to it, like I had with every other new pain over the years. I utilized my meditation practice to accept this new physical experience, as well as to navigate the suffering in my mind. I wasn't happy, but this was just the way it was going to be. I'd live a soft, low-impact life. I would do the gentlest of yoga and learn to love all the places where my body lost its tone and shape. I would avoid listening to a certain Nine Inch Nails song, so as not to get too depressed when reminded that I could no longer fuck like an animal. I would embrace sensible shoes. Maybe I would give up the expense of a car and use rideshare apps on the rare occasion I ventured out. *Hey, I thought, humans can get used to anything.*

As it turned out, I did not have to get used to that particular pain, thanks to the production of *Pain Brain*, a documentary film that "explores a new understanding of chronic pain that may provide hope to the millions who suffer."[2] An old friend of my then partner who was producing this film and knew that I experienced chronic pain invited me to be one of the participants. As an actor, I'm wary of anything unscripted (reality TV isn't great for anyone who wants to be taken seriously as an actor), but I jumped at the opportunity to be part of this when I found out what it would entail.

As a participant I would get a free session with Alan Gordon, the executive director of Pain Psychology Center in Los Angeles. Alan is a psychotherapist to the stars who developed Pain Reprocessing Therapy and coauthored *The Way Out: A Revolutionary, Scientifically Proven Approach to Healing Chronic Pain*. It's important to note that Gordon's work was heavily inspired by Dr. John Ernest Sarno, author of *Healing Back Pain: The Mind-Body Connection*. Some reviews suggest you skip Gordon's book and go straight to the source. In any case, it was Gordon I was going to see.

My partner drove me across town to Gordon's glass-walled Beverly Hills office for the filming. He was often driving me to appointments at that time. Although I appreciated him, the couple privilege I enjoyed as a spoonie became more obvious years later when we broke up. For many of us with limited spoons, a sixteen-mile solo drive through Los Angeles is enough to have us bedbound for a week, or worse. As I sat in the waiting room, I was excited to see how this therapist might be able to help me, and a little nervous of how vulnerable I might feel being observed by the filmmakers.

As they prepped me for the session, I was relieved to find out they would be in another room watching the conversation on a monitor. Once settled inside the most luxurious therapy office I've ever been in, I realized I knew Gordon's voice. I quickly came to realize that I had recently heard an interview with him on a podcast about chronic pain. I figured that this synchronicity was a good sign and got ready for the magic to happen.

We decided to focus on my degenerative disc pain because it was the most recent, most debilitating symptom. As he began to talk me through his method, my heart sunk. He was attempting to teach me basic mindfulness techniques. Trying to swallow my disappointment, I told him I had been teaching mindfulness meditation for over seven years. I wanted to cry as I started to realize this was going to be yet another list of things to manage chronic pain that I was already doing. By then I had been handed pamphlets from way too many doctors that included things like meditation, breathing techniques, and yoga. I didn't want another suggestion that could (literally) be found in a book I had written.

Being chronically ill comes with knowing way more about your ailments than many medical professionals do. For me, that can lead to a bit of an arrogant and quick-to-judge attitude if I'm not careful. It makes sense that spoonies can feel this way though. We must do our own research to find relief because of all the medical gaslighting and the gross limitations of our healthcare system. For example, most treatments I've found that actually lower my pain were not suggested

by my doctors and are not covered by my already very expensive
health insurance.

Because I knew my tendency to get annoyed and shut down in
these sorts of situations, and there was a camera pointed at me, I took
a deep a breath and vowed to myself to be open-minded and teachable. I wanted to get the most out of the experience that I could, and I
didn't want to come across as a jerk in the film or waste the filmmaker's
time. As a filmmaker myself, I knew what a few lost hours could mean.

I'm glad that I was able to pull it together and be present for what
Alan was offering. All the steps of pain reprocessing therapy (PRT)
were familiar and well-practiced for me, but his method put them all
together to create a technique that radically changed my relationship
to my chronic back pain. It interrupted the pain-fear cycle that was
making degenerative disc disease so disruptive to my life. I found that
the tools of PRT could be applied to most of my chronic pain symptoms.

Pain is a danger signal. When you are experiencing damage to
your body, this signal can be lifesaving. When you are experiencing
chronic *neuroplastic* pain, this signal can be an asshole. Neuroplastic
pain happens when the brain mistakes harmless sensations in the
body as threats and pulls a false alarm, sending the signal that danger
is imminent. Much of my pain can be considered neuroplastic.

Some indicators for neuroplastic pain include pain that arises
when you are stressed out, pain that is not connected to an injury (or
the original injury has long since healed and doesn't show up in imaging), pain that spreads and moves around, and pain that is inconsis-
tent in how and when it shows up. Ding, ding, ding, ding. Other signs
that neuroplastic pain may be present: a long list of pain symptoms,
trauma and an adverse childhood, and a leaning toward perfection-
ism, anxiety, and hypervigilance. Ding, ding, ding.

When you are experiencing this type of pain, there is likely no
damage being done to your body, but the danger signal keeps firing
anyway. This leads to the pain-fear cycle. The pain triggers the danger
signal, which creates fear, leading to scary thoughts, *What if this never*

stops? What if I'm dying?! That loop continues, even though we are not actually in physical danger, creating chronic pain.

Fibromyalgia, which researchers believe impacts the way your brain processes pain signals, has been considered a great example of neuroplastic pain.[3] This mysterious illness can cause everything from widespread body pain to chronic headaches and fatigue, to heat and cold sensitivities, to slurred speech, to sleep issues, to bladder pain. Those are just a few of my fibro symptoms. We still have much to learn about fibromyalgia and the hellscape of pain it delivers. One recent study suggests it doesn't originate in the brain but is actually an auto-immune disease.[4] There is also new research with promising data showing that fibromyalgia could be connected to alterations in gut biome.[5] It may turn out that advancements in medical science show that fibro pain isn't neuroplastic and that the danger alarms are accurate. That would be a miracle if it led to a cure, but in the meantime, treating fibro pain as neuroplastic can be incredibly helpful.

Approaching fibro pain as a faulty alarm system going haywire *does not mean your fibro pain isn't real or that relief is as simple as a single method.* A fibro flare-up can feel like you are on the verge of death. There are so many kinds of pain all at the same time, which means tons of danger signals firing. Even on a day without an active flare-up, the number of symptoms can be staggering. But medically and anatomically speaking, no physical damage is actually being done at the points that are in pain. (Psychological pain is another story.)

This non-damaging pain can also originate from an injury. For example, I was in a car accident in 2002 and had some slight soft tissue damage to my right shoulder. For years afterward anytime I was stressed or upset, that shoulder would start hurting terribly, even though there was no visible damage. My brain, already wired to send all kinds of unnecessary pain signals (thanks, fibromyalgia), just kept on sending those asshole signals.

PRT uses mindfulness to help bring curiosity and acceptance to neuroplastic pain, which allows you to identify it as just a sensation (e.g., pressure, tingling, heat) rather than label it pain. Next, to reframe the sensations as not dangerous, safety reappraisal is introduced. In the case of my lingering shoulder pain I might say, *My shoulder has a contraction and pinching sensation, but I know there is nothing wrong with the muscles and joints of my shoulder. My brain is just confused right now.* This message cuts the danger signal short and gives your brain a different story to chew on. Then you bring in a little positive self-talk in the form of some humor or an easy breezy attitude. *My brain is such a silly goose!* This isn't about some sort of toxic positivity or downplaying your experience in a condescending way. The positive affect induction just helps lighten things up so that your brain is more open to being retrained.

To be very, very clear, the way I use and suggest this method is not denying that your pain exists. Your pain is real. Why the hell would you be spending time learning some technique to deal with it if it weren't? I know I wouldn't have spent countless hours and dollars on seeking solutions for something that wasn't real. It's also important to state that while PRT has been shown to be quite effective, that doesn't mean it will be a match for everyone. It is a match for me, for *some* pain.[6] Partly because, given my background in meditation, I was an ideal candidate for this method.

Part of what had made the lower back pain so unbearable was that I was scared something was terribly wrong. That fear of actual damage being done made it hard for me to find equanimity through meditation the way I had been able to with other chronic pain. For example, once I found out that what I thought were continued chronic urinary tract infections was actually interstitial cystitis, it became easy to put my meditation practice into action. It was still uncomfortable, but without the fear of serious infection, it was no longer overwhelming or debilitating. When I was diagnosed with degenerative disc disease, I was also a little gun-shy when it came to having too much equanimity with pain. A few years earlier my ability to deconstruct pain with meditation had kept me from recognizing that I had a serious health issue that required medical attention, which landed me in the ER. Some pain is causing damage. You need to be able to discern what is actually dangerous, and sometimes we need more than our own opinion.

I learned that having too much acceptance with pain can be dangerous. When I started meditating, I was a bit of a masochist. As if I didn't already have enough pain to meditate on, I would do things like hold my arms out to the side for an hourlong sit, focus on the most painful sensations every time I meditated, or sit for four hours at a time without moving. I thought I was so hardcore. My chronic pain also gave me endless material to practice on, and I was doing this with painful emotions too. The idea was that I would no longer experience pain as pain, but rather as just impermanent sensations arising and passing. I got quite good at deconstructing pain and could tolerate high levels without a lot of suffering. By the time I had a series of health crises that culminated in a bleeding stomach and a hospital stay, I had gotten a little too good at this and missed the actual danger signals that my body was sending. I then needed to take some time to reacquaint myself with pain as pain. I still like an occasional four-hour meditation, but I'm much gentler with my body now. I don't regret the path I was on, as it was fruitful in all kinds of ways, and today I'm way more attuned to the difference between pain that is not really a problem and pain that might be causing my body real damage.

Technically, degenerative disk disease *is* slowly causing damage, but it's not an emergency. I was, and still am, far from the type of degeneration that is cause for concern. This meant I could let go of the idea that something was terribly wrong. Before I even got out of the fancy office and into the car, I was already putting PRT to work. I opted for these safety reappraisal phrases: *There is no damage being done. There is no danger. I am safe.* Each time I felt that pain in the week following the session, I interrupted my brain from sending the danger signal with those words. I was relentless. Again, the years of meditation gave me an advantage, and I'm not sure I would have been able to have such resolve without all that practice of concentration, sensory clarity, and acceptance. Nonetheless, after that one PRT session, I never experienced the degenerative disc symptoms in the same way again.

Putting together the tools of mindfulness, safety reappraisal, and positive affect has become a go-to pain management technique for me, and in turn for many of my trauma-resolution clients, who almost all have some sort of chronic neuroplastic pain. Mindfulness alone had been working fairly well to manage my pain, but hijacking those faulty danger signals in such a simple, specific, and intentional way increased the relief and my quality of life. It's also been incredibly rewarding to see the same for people who I've shared the techniques with.

Anxiety and fatigue can also be considered danger signals. Anxiety is a hyper-aroused nervous system response, and fatigue is a hypo-aroused response. In my early life, the flight energy of anxiety and the freeze energy of fatigue helped me survive. But as I cultivated a safe and stable life for myself as an adult, my brain still thought it needed to trigger these embodied emergency responses, leading to a chronic state of being wired and tired. One foot on the gas and one on the brake. My undiagnosed ADHD and autism also led to being anxious and burned out much of the time. Thinking of these C-PTSD- and neurodivergent-related issues as neuroplastic pain and using PRT to address them has been a huge help in navigating and reducing them.

My back still fucking hurts, but in the ways it always has, and I manage that pain with much success through a combination of all the things that work for me. As for the pain that came upon me while I was naked in front of a camera, the disc pain, it's gone. That mind control shit worked. I never feel it anymore, even when I fuck like an animal or wear nonsense shoes (which I wear less often since coming out as non-binary, embracing my gender expression, and rediscovering the euphoria of Dr. Martens and loafers). The interesting thing is that the sensation my brain was deciphering as pain is probably still present, I just don't notice it now that there is no danger signal being sent. I find that to be strange and wonderful. We really can change our brain, and that means we can change so much of our experience as humans. The possibilities are endless.

The Feast

When you are starving, breadcrumbs are a feast.
Licking your fingerprints, bringing the mouse's meal to your lips.
Saying *thank you* and *please*,
pushing down the feral hunger growing in the growl of your guts with
a performance of polite.

At age fourteen, I sat in my adult boyfriend's parked car
as he shamed me for every sound my concave stomach made
and every long silence I could not fill with my child's voice:
What is wrong with you?

He must have forgotten how only months before, cruel laughter in his
throat, he said:
Your belly is cute. Just don't gain any weight.

He must have forgotten that

I spoke
too loud
about
things that
he didn't even care about.

He bombed me with love until I grew accustomed to the feeling of
fullness
from him warming my hands on a snowy east coast day
from notes full of x's and o's
from mixtapes of dangerously obsessive love songs
from attention, undivided and endless.

Once I trusted the taste of being satiated
he told me I had eaten too much:

selfish
arrogant
greedy—and put me on a crash diet.

Starved and dismantled, I ran from him
filling my hands and pockets and mouth with anything in sight,
and he tracked me like a bloodhound
masked in sweetness to say:

I have everything you need
Put down that bread
Open your lips, spit out that bite
Let me back in.

He came back in incessantly,
feeding me just a little less each time.
teaching me how to subsist with smaller portions
until I needed nearly nothing.

Finally, my hollowed reflection in the window of a storefront scared
me awake
my feral overtook my polite

I dropped his empty plate
didn't look back to see it shatter

Then I ate and ate and ate.

And This Is ADHD

I want to tell you about all the things I didn't know were symptoms of ADHD. I want to list them and write a quippy paragraph about each one. Instead, I take a moment to confirm that I'm remembering correctly that both overplanning *and* underplanning are symptoms and I get lost in the Google forest and the big bad time-blindness wolf invites me into a few hours of research on a myriad of things.

Somehow, I end up on the phone with my insurance company asking them if they will cover my Botox treatments that reduce my chronic tension headaches. I don't tell them that I like the way it lifts my eyes, making me look less tired. Fatigue makes me look droopy. They say I need a CPT code from my doctor. I can't follow the instructions, even though it's just one simple sentence. I cannot process this information. *You'll need to call us back with a CPT code.* It sounds like *Wah Wha Wha Wha code.* I ask again, as I manage the emotional dysregulation that always shows up when I call my insurance company. How many times has *This call may be recorded for quality and training purposes* caught me crying? I couldn't begin to guess.

I ask them to email the instructions. *Was my tone irritated and condescending? Am I being the most annoying person in the world?* Neutral tone. Neutral tone. No, they will not email me because all they need is the CPT code. I am trying to retain this, *C as in Cat P as in Paul T as in Tom* (I'm too overwhelmed managing my tone and my emotions to change P to *Paula* and T to *Tamara.* I am failing at being a feminist). *No,* they say, *C as in Cat P as in Paul T as in Tom*. I don't say, *That is what I just said*, because it's entirely possible that I said something else. I'll get that code. I'll get back to them. I'm getting a headache. I don't have a neurologist. *What was my old neurologist's name? I'll never find it. Should I search my old inboxes? No, I'll never find it.*

Why aren't I more organized? He is the one who diagnosed me with chronic tension headaches and migraines, and now he is lost to me forever. I need to find a neurologist. Now. I'm searching through names. Which one should I call? What if I choose the wrong one? What if they don't believe me about my pain? What if they tell my insurance company that I don't have chronic tension headaches and migraines and that I don't need Botox?

This has become a very important decision and I am paralyzed by choice paralysis. I don't call anyone. I give up on that task and try to remember what I was doing. What I *am* doing is biting at my cuticles and curling my toes into my shoes repeatedly. My fresh manicure was a temporary cure for the abuse of my cuticles, and now I am fucking it up. I switch to scratching my head and feeling for little bumps to pick from my back.

These are but a few of my stims and but a few of the places my ADHD overlaps with my autism. AuDHD all day, baby! My clothing is uncomfortable and I take a trip down memory lane to being an undiagnosed AuDHD kid with sensory processing disorder who was always ripping my clothes off because they felt *taggy* or itchy or too tight or too soft. I come back from my travels to days gone by and I realize I'm also too cold, but if I change my clothes I'll walk by the bathroom and then I'll start plucking my chin hairs and get stuck in the mirror for thirty minutes. If I turn off the air conditioner I'll just get too hot. I never seem to feel just right. Just call me Jess "Goldilocks" Graham. Now I feel hungry. My stomach growls like a big old papa bear. I forgot to eat lunch. I have an almost full liter of water in front of me, but I haven't taken a sip in hours. Shit, it's been hours. I have to leave the house at five to be on time to my acting class. I rush to class every single week. I don't want to be late—again. I'll have to leave early from class because I have to get up early tomorrow and it takes me hours to wind down after the stimuli of class. Let's be honest, even if I come home early I won't put myself to bed on time. I stay up late. I always have. I don't see clients until 11 a.m. for a reason, which is that I stay up late.

I'm nauseous. I waited too long to eat. Now the texture of my lunch will be even more disgusting. I'm disgusted with this soup and with these crackers. They are no longer safe foods, and so I eat ice cream instead. I'm engaging in addictive behaviors with sugar, just like I used to do with alcohol. I told myself not to buy the multiple pints of vegan ice cream because if I had the multiple pints of ice cream I would eat the multiple pints of vegan ice cream within seventy-two hours. Then would come the guilt. But I did buy the ice cream and right now the sugar feels great. Ice cream is always a safe food, thank you, Baby Jesus.

A terrible thought. The kind I get after lunch with a new friend. Did I share too much? Will I be rejected by you, my reader, for giving you this glimpse into what it's like on the days I take off from my Adderall so that I don't build up a tolerance? Will I be criticized for not using all my meditative tools to manage my neurodivergent brain? Maybe I'll never let you read this. Nah, fuck that. Rejection sensitive dysphoria kept me in hiding for far too long and I'm no little pig, even if I have hairs on my chinny chin chin. I blew that house down myself a long time ago. I have superpowers. I have courage and resilience. I'm not just impulsive, I'm spontaneous! I don't just share too much, I spark intriguing conversations! I don't just have distractibility, I have hyperfocus! I don't just have fatigue, I have high energy! Also, us ADHD folks are creative as fuck. Time to wash that load of laundry for a third time since it got mildew scented from sitting for too long again. Wheeeeeee.

The Wrongness
and the Goodness

Here where productivity is seen as a sign of self-worth and hustle culture is celebrated. Here where the dream of the American Dream lulls us to sleep while the rich get richer. Here where the world is built for the able-bodied and the neurotypical. Here where wellness is a multi-trillion-dollar industry and quality mental healthcare is a luxury. Here where the education system has cracks all over and underneath those there's more. Here where tech gods create screens as addictive as oxycontin but don't let their kids use them. Here where executive disfunction is mislabeled as lazy. Here where we talk around what we really mean, translating every interaction into corporate email speak. Here where the soothing regenerative experience of nature is replaced by cubicles and classrooms and burnout binges of reality TV. Here where rest has been forgotten in the mad dance of capitalism and the bottom line. Here where brains like mine travel to the beat of a different drum than most.

It was there, in that reality, that my neurodivergence was discovered. But that reality shifted when I was given the gift of the truth—a relative truth—about myself. The labels we wear, including our age, gender, and even species, are clothing that allows us to make sense of a mystery too vast to begin to comprehend. Some of the labels we claim as ours, or have thrust upon us, are ill-fitted, covered in tags that itch, and sewn of fabric made of microfiber. Some labels set us free, naked as we came. The labels of Autism and Attention Deficit/Hyperactivity Disorder (which can be shortened to AuDHD) are the latter garment for me. My diagnosis, a welcome surprise, still celebrated to this day.

The ADHD diagnosis came first, then the autism diagnosis three years later. I must confess I once was unable to celebrate the diagnosis of ADHD when it was given to others. Instead, I judged, and then I envied. When my sister was prescribed little blue pills for ADHD, which left her working harder than her classmates at university, I railed against it. *That is just legal speed. You should just meditate. You are going to get addicted.* As the eldest, my opinion held great sway, but my little sister did not bend to my will this time. She used the medicine she needed, the medicine that allowed her mind to quiet and focus, the medicine that her doctor prescribed. How absurd that I thought I knew better. How hilarious that I didn't recognize that we shared neurodivergence. How grateful I am that she didn't obey and now, though it makes her giggle, that she doesn't judge or lecture me. She didn't get addicted, and she meditates daily. She uses other methods to treat her symptoms now, and she is thriving. That sweet sister of mine went on to get a master's in education and is top of her field, abroad, living, as she says, a life beyond her wildest dreams.

After the days of judgment and righteousness ended, I found myself in the time of envy. Going undiagnosed into my forties, and incessant pain, left me in a perpetual state of burnout. What had been bouts of chronic fatigue since childhood evolved into years of unending and life-force-draining exhaustion. I did not know that fatigue is a common symptom of ADHD. Nor did I know that my foggy brain was partly due to neurodivergence. At this peak state of neurodivergent burnout, I had a friend who had been diagnosed with ADHD late in life. She told me of her new lease on life now that she was medicated and aware of what interventions she could employ to address her symptoms. My happiness for her was not without envy. What she described as her symptoms overlapped with mine.

The battle to go to bed before the morning news anchors came on. The impulsivity. The clutter, unfolded laundry, dirty dishes, full inboxes, unopened mail. The debt. The piles of papers. The feeling of never being able to catch up, of always being behind. The feeling that no matter how hard I worked, or how much I achieved, it was never quite enough. The wondering why after so many years of meditation and unwinding and resolution of trauma, there was still the subtle sense, deep in the gut, that I was marked with wrongness. And the deep, deep fatigue. We both knew these struggles, but unlike my friend, I had no diagnosis to explain them, and no medication to alleviate them. I didn't consider even once that I too might be diagnosable, but oh how I wished I could get the relief she enjoyed.

There were other symptoms that I had wrestled to be relieved of—masking to survive, fit in, be loved. Before my meltdowns were met with harsh words or worse, I howled and thrashed like a wolf child trapped in domesticated hell. Before I learned to swallow the suffering to be polite, I was known to get up from my seat and walk out of a restaurant before ordering if the lights weren't quite right or the acoustics of the room were troubling. Before I was chided by a boyfriend for being a *picky* eater and obeyed his instructions, I could suddenly hate eggs, or other foods with textures I couldn't abide, for years at a time. Before I was shamed by a colleague for the volume of my voice during a meeting, my voice boomed and echoed. Before I was told to walk *normally* for years on end by everyone from partners to friends to film directors, my stride was strange and inimitable. Before I decided that my fidgeting, stimming, self-soothing, and excessive grooming were to be meditated out of me, I was in shameless and constant movement, a full expression of release, an internal dance set free. These can all be found at the intersection of ADHD and autism, and in my case they are.

These *symptoms* have been slowly reframed and unshamed, masks torn asunder, since I was given the gift of a good diagnosis. A friend and creative kindred once said, *A good diagnosis can change your life.* This seems to be true. A wave of relief flooded my life when I was told I had ADHD. I no longer felt drowned by a murky feeling of wrongness in being me, and instead I was awash with the crystal clear goodness of self-compassion and understanding. The autism diagnosis has been more of a tsunami, the waters of relief mixed with grief. I am still coming to understand how deep the masks go, and some days I wonder if I ever will.

Before the relief, I lived in envy and judgment, when I decided that I too was deserving of psychiatric care. Why hadn't I sought that support sooner? Because my work was to help others find resolution with the harmful imprints of their lives, because I could meditate for hours on end, because I was a meditation *teacher*, because I believed that I was one rotation around the trauma recovery wheel from no longer feeling that wrongness. Because I didn't have much faith in the field made famous by white men whom we call *fathers of psychiatry.*

In fact, I had not seen a psychiatrist since I was twenty years old when, in a matter of one weekend, a very close and deeply loved family member attempted suicide and I found out I was pregnant with a child I knew I could not birth. It was too much for my nervous system, already stuck in an emergency response since before the inauguration of Reagan. I ran to the comfort of a crisis center, but I didn't say the words that called for a locked latch, limited linens, and the heavy door opening every fifteen minutes. I didn't want to die, but life had me in headlock and I yelled uncle. They medicated me, after I promised, cross my heart and hope to die, that the fetus would not be taking up residence inside me for more than a few weeks. They sent me on my way with the number of a low-cost clinic and a week's supply of happy pills.

The psychiatrist who saw me later that week was a tiny terror behind a giant desk in a dark room. She shamed me for being non-monogamous, saying she couldn't help me and neither could the therapist if I kept my boyfriend and my girlfriend. Her eyes were angry lasers looking at my large Dunkin' Donuts coffee, saying *all that caffeine, no wonder you are depressed and anxious. And the sugar!* She put me on Effexor, and when I complained of the side effects (hearing laugher and mocking voices that were not there, crushing waves of paranoia, bulging eyes that wouldn't shut at night) and told her I'd no longer take it, she yelled words that I'll never forget: *You're going to be banging on my door, begging for me to put you back on it.* I never saw her door again. Although I now have respected colleagues and a beloved client who are physiatrists, after that experience I soured on seeking psychiatric care for two decades.

Then one evening, lost in hyperfixated research of random topics stemming from other random topics, I came across a list of symptoms of ADHD in women and those socialized as women. As I read, the image of a bright green check mark appeared in my mind for every symptom. Then I promptly *forgot*. The kind of forgetting that comes on like a fast-moving fever, burning off the cool splash of clarity. Forgetting that depends on denial. Forgetting that whispers, *Look away, look away, nothing to see here, dear.* It seemed to me that most anything on that list could be explained away by the complexities of childhood trauma anyway.

Some fragment of clear, cool clarity survived the denial, and I dared to imagine that perhaps some of what had followed me through life was not strictly C-PTSD. I had, after all, made great strides in changing my nervous system, and much had improved. Could it be that the wrongness was not based on a body that had been flash-frozen with fight and flight when it was small? This fatigue, disorganization, procrastination, and not-enoughness—what if a doctor who diagnosed from the *DSM* could explain? What if it didn't need to be this hard?

First there was a woman who, during our virtual sessions, never looked up at her screen as she typed furiously and asked again and again, *And how is your sleep?* I listed my symptoms, trying to be brief, knowing that many stop listening when the list is too long. I told her that I could not tolerate the numb clit of SSRIs or the suicidal ideation of SNRIs. Though she never knew the color of my eyes, she saw a path to wellness for me with the norepinephrine–dopamine reuptake inhibitor Wellbutrin. I love to say I love that drug. I love to say it to people who think a meditation teacher can lean toward psychedelics but never toward pharmaceuticals. I like to disrupt beliefs based on what is *spiritual* and what is not.

Wellbutrin was magical, giving me the first sustained energy I had felt in years and making undone tasks seem to do themselves. Alas the thrill was dimmed and the dose increased after a few weeks. The doctor who I could only contact on an app soon grew bored with my questions and requests, and her replies came slow and short. This NDRI still supports me, so I am grateful for her instinct, but making me feel seen and heard was not her strong suit.

I did not cease my seeking, and found myself in the virtual office of a young psychiatric nurse practitioner. I could hear his dog bark in the background and saw colorful art on his walls, and he saw and heard me. He saw that I was dedicated to my mental health. He heard me say that I was tired all the time and that I could never seem to feel caught up on life. After three sessions he asked, *Have you ever been on a stimulant? Let's assess you for ADHD.* The night of the green check marks came flooding back, from forgotten to fresh. *Yes, let's do that, please.* With the remembering, a fragment started to shine and spread.

Weeks prior I had hired a life coach who had found her way to my TikTok "For You" page (TikTok is yet another thing I love to love out loud, without a care for any judgment). She was an *ADHD coach*. I hired her with no intention of utilizing her specific skillset, but rather because I liked her social media personality. I came to find that her online persona was authentic, which made me like her even more. We did not speak about neurodivergence, as far as I recall, until I shared the news that I was to be assessed. She gave me a knowing look and her expressive eyebrows and joyful smile said, *Yeah, obviously you are neurodivergent, why do you think I found my way to your TikTok For You page?* That algorithm is something else, I tell you. She told me books to read and tools to use as I awaited my diagnosis.

The diagnosis came like spring after the longest winter, like the puzzle piece that was lost until you moved house and did a deep clean, like an answered prayer you didn't know you were praying, like ice-cold Gatorade when you are hungover and have no air-conditioning and it's ninety-nine degrees. It came like a good diagnosis because it was.

Goodness replaced wrongness almost instantaneously. I thought I knew self-compassion. And I did, but I also knew that seed of wrong inside my gut. Entering streams, riding bulls, and the freedom from much suffering had not dislodged what was planted in my navel. The diagnosis of ADHD didn't remove the seedling, it transmuted it into something that could grow and bloom. That blooming was compassion, understanding, relief, and self-discovery. That blooming was permission, finally granted, to be who I am without apology. That blooming was a homecoming, by way of understanding that I could no longer shove myself into the home that *here* told me was mine. I could see why here had been so hard to be. It wasn't a moral failing, or the remnants of trauma, or a case of just needing to try harder, better, more. The truth revealed. Here had not been built for me.

World building as I go, these are the things that were allowed to unfold:

I cut my hair. How long it had grown in my trying to be *a girl* who my partners would kneel before, ring in hand, and claim as their own. How long it had grown as I protected my heart from half-truths and lights fueled by gas. Looking at the pile of brown strands next to the silver shears on the stylist's table, I saw the past and walked away.

I said my last goodbye to that kind of partner. Done with the wound of being unchosen being opened again and again. Done with the gendering and gender roles. I claimed myself. Not *a girl*. Not exactly a woman. Certainly not a man. Outside the binary, just as I had always been.

I started writing poetry and creative nonfiction again. I made a beautiful home just for me and my tiny scruffy dog. I enjoyed better health. I got angry and didn't bury it in my joints and muscles. I swam naked under the stars in Mexico. I went back to acting class. I bought a white car, drove it right off the lot, knowing I was worthy of safety and that new car smell. I embraced the single life and became my own boyfriend. I became social again. I made forever friends who cooked me steaks when I was sad and took me to church.

Never religious, I vetted a church and got baptized when they came back clean of hate and bigotry. I let Jesus love me. I let loved ones love me. I fell in love with Ireland and drove across the Emerald Isle with my littlest sister in the passenger seat. I read more novels. I was able to go to a theme park with my family without melting down from stimuli. I found out I actually love theme parks after thinking I hated them for years. I started having fun. I laughed out loud daily. I felt a joy that had always been there, just beneath a thick layer of foggy ice. I fell in love with being me.

This unfolding was in big part due to the diagnosis and understanding of myself. It was also because of how well I've done on the medications I was prescribed. The first time I took Adderall felt like being two weeks into a silent meditation retreat, or the effects of two hours of meditation a day. Peaceful, focused, awake. My dopamine-hungry brain is now fed. Wellbutrin, Adderall, and most recently low-dose naltrexone, which not only treats my chronic pain but seems to be having a positive impact on negative symptoms of the ADHD. This combination of big pharma offerings has freed me from a lifetime of exhaustion, allowed me to enjoy experiences that previously caused overstimulation, given me the ability to focus my mind without hours of daily meditation, and made me a hell of a lot happier.

These drugs work for me. My life is easier. That ease makes way for more joy and less effort. I efforted for as long as I can remember, trying to keep up with some imaginary idea of who I was supposed to be and what I was supposed to accomplish. I measured myself against

Silicon Valley bros and Mark Wahlberg–style daily routines. I couldn't see how much I had actually accomplished and against what odds. I found creative ways to function at a fairly high level in many areas of my life, and the ADHD diagnosis helped me give myself some credit and appreciation. I stopped judging the way I did things, and trying to conform to some neurotypical standard, and instead started celebrating and utilizing my divergent way of moving through the world. As much as that diagnosis changed my life, it was only the beginning of my neurodivergent adventure.

The night I came across the list for ADHD, I had been watching videos about autism being diagnosed late in life. TikTok had fed me these videos, evidently knowing more about me than I did at the time. There was a resonance deep inside me as I watched people share their stories of being autistic in an allistic world. However, I immediately started gaslighting myself. I picked out the few things that I didn't relate to and decided that everything else was just a coincidence. I did ask a few people close to me if they thought I might be autistic, consensus was no. Most folks think of Dustin Hoffman's character in *Rain Man* or children with very high support needs when they hear the word *autism*. None of my doctors or therapists noticed the signs in me either, and when I got the ADHD diagnosis, I pinned all my neurodivergent qualities to that, C-PTSD, and aspects of chronic illness.

A few years passed and I continued to unmask my ADHD. I began to notice how much of myself I had been hiding away under those masks. My masking went much deeper than I had first thought, and I was bone-tired from keeping up the many façades. Leaving that bad relationship, coming out as non-binary, and all the new awareness of what I needed and how I wanted to express energized me, but I knew there was more to shed and to claim. The more I became myself, the more of myself I wanted to bring out of hiding. I wasn't sure that ADHD could explain everything I felt bubbling under the surface of my attempts to belong. There was more of me, and I could hear them asking to be seen, understood, and loved.

After a series of in-depth self-assessment tests came back showing a high likelihood of autism, I decided to get a formal assessment from a professional. Over the course of six weeks, I met with a gentle, warm, and kind-eyed psychologist named Dr. Lee who specialized in adult autism diagnosis. She asked questions and I answered them, that was it. These simple interviews were deceptively powerful and profound. Foundations and pillars of my personality, decades old, began to tremble and quake as I talked about my history of sensory processing challenges, confusing social and workplace interactions, and all the ways I had managed and controlled even the most basic movements of my body so as to appear *normal*. How, no matter how much effort I made, I still felt that sense of wrongness in just being me.

I shared about the trials and tribulations of eye contact; how much was not enough, and how much was too much? We spent more than a session talking about which textures, sounds, touches, and sights I enjoyed, and which made me deeply uncomfortable. I told her how I had practiced for years to be able to put myself in someone else's shoes and how everyday empathy didn't come naturally to me unless the roles were clearly defined. With my clients or others who look to me as a teacher or guide, I am easily empathic. But in other, less defined relationships, it can take more effort. She asked me if I had special interests and I shared that sex, psychology, spirituality, and film and theater have been my passions, and even obsessions, since I was a small child. Dr. Lee started to say, at least once a session, *That's not uncommon for autistic people.* As we progressed, and before getting the diagnosis, I started to experience shifts.

About two weeks into the assessment, I had a social gathering at my house. I always prefer social interactions that involve activities, or that I'm hosting. Activities, such as a game night or dancing, give me something to focus on and help me understand how to interact. If I'm hosting, I can focus on playing the role of host. Still, even with a defined role or activity, social interaction can be overstimulating and leave me burnt out for days, or even weeks. After learning more about myself through the questions Dr. Lee had been asking me, I decided to try an experiment. I would just be myself, completely, throwing asunder all masks for the evening.

The relief was undeniable. I felt free and joyful as I allowed my interactions with friends to be natural and organic, unafraid of being perceived as abnormal. I didn't manage the way I moved my body, the expressions on my face, or the sounds that I made. I talked about the things that interest me and trusted that if someone was ready to change the subject, they would let me know. I was shocked to realize how much of myself I normally hid, and how good it felt to be out in the open. I didn't spend precious energy (or spoons) masking and I accounted for my sensitivities, which meant I didn't end up burnt out and overstimulated. What unfolded that night was a paradigm shift that is still very much underway. I have been masking so much of myself for so long. It will take time to understand all the ways I've pretended to be other than what I am. I am patient with myself as I unlearn all the false versions of me.

At the end of the six-week assessment, I wasn't sure what she would say. As much as it seemed glaringly obvious that I was a high masking autistic, I, like many others, still thought the traits had to be more extreme to qualify me for an autism diagnosis. As we neared the middle of our final session, Dr. Lee looked at me with her kind eyes and asked if there was anything I needed before she gave me the diagnosis. I asked for a moment to take a deep breath and then said, *Lay it on me, Dr. Lee.* When I heard the words *Jess, you are autistic*, I instantly began to cry. As she outlined how she had arrived at the diagnosis and the ways C-PTSD and ADHD do and don't overlap with autism, I continued to weep. Those tears were the salty waters of grief and relief, long held under my striving to get rid of the wrongness.

The truth is there is nothing wrong with me. Yes, I'll continue to refine the human that is me to be kinder to myself and others, to be freer and more creative in my expression, to be of greater service and to inspire less suffering wherever I can. I'll keep working on bringing goodness to the world, but without the belief that wrongness infuses my very being. Knowing that I am autistic doesn't solve every challenge that arises, but understanding this about myself has decreased many challenges and increased my well-being.

With this growing understanding of how I operate, I can now give myself, or request, accommodations as needed. I got myself earplugs that allow for conversation while blocking out other sounds that can overwhelm me. I can ask a friend to adjust the lights, or volume of music, when I'm feeling overstimulated. I share that I'm autistic with new people in my life and give them information that creates more intimacy and less confusion in our interactions. I give myself lots of time alone, now understanding that just the experience of being perceived by another human can be a lot for me to navigate. Relief continues to arrive as I get to know myself through the lens of autism.

There is also much to grieve. How different my life might have been if I had this information earlier. How many close friendships might not have ended due to misunderstandings that could have easily been avoided. I likely wouldn't have allowed myself to be controlled by abusive partners who didn't approve of my sensitivities and stims if I hadn't been judging them myself. Would I have experienced less chronic pain if I wasn't chronically policing myself in every interaction? If I hadn't carried the unexplainable feelings of wrong throughout my life, I may have experienced more feelings of good. As it is, I am making up for lost time, tapping the wellspring of goodness, drinking my fill.

The relief and grief keep coming in waves as I orient to this new world I've found myself in. Shortly after being diagnosed, I made a TikTok video describing receiving an autism diagnosis late in life. I said that it's like getting into a spaceship and going to a planet where all the physics are different and you don't understand anything at all, and yet everything makes sense. I'm starting to get my balance, and as I make sense of this strange land, I'm not as much of a stranger to myself. I'm falling more in love with the goodness of being me.

I don't consider my autism and ADHD to be problems that need solving. I don't consider myself to be a problem to solve anymore. This means I don't work so hard. I've been released from the endless effort of adapting to what is considered correct or normal.

I let life be easier now. It's okay to let life be easier.

Here I am free.

Here where I say fuck hustle culture. Here where my bottom line is based on joy. Here where I'm doing enough, I have enough, I am enough. Here where self-compassion is cellular deep. Here where I sweep up the ashes of all the masks I've worn. Here where I don't eat eggs unless I want to and don't let anyone tell me who to be. Here where what were once limitations are now seen as superpowers. Here where the square of atypical has broken apart into glistening fragments of possibility.

Here where the beat of my drum is loud and clear and mine to shamelessly share.

Love in the Time of Hemorrhoids

There is a problem with my shit. Or rather with my experience of shitting. I can go from peeing from my ass to so blocked up I have to go to the ER. I've had shit problems since I was a kid. I have an incredibly vivid memory of *almost* making it to the toilet with some explosive diarrhea when I was six. Some of it made it in the bowl, but my anus must have been on fan mode, because there was a spray of shit all over the tank, the wall, the side of the bathtub, and the floor. I don't think I was old enough to be embarrassed exactly, maybe more concerned about how my mother would react to the brown-splattered bathroom, which she already struggled to keep clean along with taking care of three kids and an alcoholic husband.

Later when I was twelve and went to the best hippie school this side of the 1970s, I had another incident that I can say with full confidence was embarrassing. My poor little constipated guts finally let loose a massive and rock-hard shit during school one day. The bathroom was *in* the classroom. It was already mortifying enough that I had to poop at school, but when the toilet, that was probably installed before 1970, got clogged and overflowed out into the classroom, that was a whole new realm of humiliation. These are only two of many bowel-related memories. It occurs to me that people who don't have problems with shitting probably also don't have a catalog of *that time when I took a shit* stories.

Try as I might to manage it, and I do try, I continue to have flare-ups of the gastrointestinal variety. When I recently messaged my GI doctor with the new and increased symptoms I've been experiencing, whatever I said, and the fact that my grandfather died from Crohn's disease, triggered a swift response and a nearly immediate scheduling for an endoscopy and colonoscopy. In layperson's terms, they are going to stick one camera way up my ass and another down my throat into my stomach. This will require anesthesia and twenty-four-hour supervision afterward. In my opinion it will also require some Valium or Xanax because I have a great fear of being conscious but unable to speak or move while under anesthesia. Also because anesthesia always makes me wake up sobbing, and honestly, I'd like to just pop a pill rather than use all my *tools* to work through it.

When receiving a procedure, such as the delightful one I will soon experience, you need a friend or family member to pick you up. It can't be an Uber. I've been single for almost two years, and this is the first time I've felt sad about it. I love being single. After eleven years in an emotionally exhausting and at times downright abusive relationship (and only one year single before that since I was fourteen), I like my space, time, and energy to be mine alone. So there aren't a lot of people who I'd like to pick me up post–spit roast by alien probes. If it's anything like the other times I've had these kinds of procedures, or really anything medical involving needing a driver afterward, I will be feeling incredibly vulnerable and raw skinned (with a sore throat and ass) when they roll me out in my white paper gown. I have no family nearby, and some of my closest and oldest friends don't live near me either. While I do have wonderful friends, one of whom will pick me up post-procedure, this is a time when a partner would really fit the bill. If I'm in a bad flare-up (or need to be picked up at the medical clinic), I don't want to hang out with someone who I don't know very, very well. Or who I feel the need to impress with clothing that doesn't involve elastic waistbands and oversized sweatshirts.

Having a partner as a chronically ill person can be such a huge support in a multitude of ways, someone to take you to invasive procedures being just one. A past partner of mine was the first person to acknowledge (and help me realize) that I have chronic pain. He witnessed the way I protected certain parts of my body and how often I took Advil. We lived together, so he saw how much pain I was in every morning when I woke up and how I struggled to find foods that wouldn't exacerbate my symptoms. He also experienced chronic pain, so that added to his ability to see what was going on with me, as well as his capacity for compassion. I asked another partner, from my early twenties, if she remembered me being in pain all the time. Her main memory was that she gave me massages nearly every day. She gave damn good massages, which makes her swoon-worthy to spoonie.

Co-regulation with a partner can have a major positive impact on my mental and emotional state related to my illnesses. In most of my relationships I wanted tons of physical connection. If I feel safe and comfortable with someone, I can cuddle and snuggle for hours (though if I'm in a lot of pain it needs to be done strategically). Connecting body to body can calm the fight/flight/freeze response that gets activated with chronic pain. A calmed nervous system and embodied sense of safety tend to lead to less pain, or at least less distress associated with the pain. Of course, co-regulation can happen with platonic friends, or even with someone I'm dating. During a particularly stressful time in my life, I briefly dated a lovely young man who I would ask to just lay on top of me for fifteen minutes to give me some co-regulation. We weren't in a committed relationship, but you don't have to be to get that need met.

A good partner who you feel comfortable and safe being with in the messiness of chronic illness can be a godsend. They see the battles you win and the battles you lose. They know, to the degree that they are able, what you are experiencing day-to-day. They don't make silly or hurtful comments about your health and body like those who don't know you so well can unintentionally do. They are there when you

wake up on a bad pain morning and there when you go to bed celebrating a decrease in symptoms. They love you, care for you, and see
you as more than your illness. Being seen, known, accepted, and loved
by someone who you also like to have orgasms with can do wonders
for quality of life.

There's also the benefit of having a two-income household when
you are partnered. That comes in handy when my medical costs ask
me to tithe more than an evangelical megachurch. My rent alone
doubled when I left my last relationship. Living together also, ideally,
means splitting the household duties, though the household duties
decreased when I became single this last time as I was only cleaning
for one. That wasn't always the case in other relationships though.
Actually, for the most part my partners and I did a pretty good job
of sharing the load and divvying up chores. One thing I did get in
my last relationship was someone willing to drive almost every time
we went somewhere together. In fact, there were plenty of times he
drove me somewhere he *wasn't* going, including to a book signing 400
miles from where we lived. The stimuli and physical impact of driving can take quite a toll on me, so that made a big difference for my
overall well-being. Another way that relationship was supportive to
living well with chronic conditions was that it was non-monogamous
a majority of the time.

Ethical non-monogamy (ENM) isn't right for everyone. It might
make things worse healthwise if it causes regular conflict, and navigating and maintaining multiple relationships can cost a lot of spoons. If
ENM is without thought and mindfulness or isn't actually ethical but
instead abusive (been there), it's not going to be helpful. And yet ENM
done well can be an excellent option for chronically ill folks and their
partners. Being sick means needing help—sometimes a lot more help
than one person can offer. A ride to the doctor, a shoulder to soak with
snot and tears, or someone to help you remember to take your meds
or do your physical therapy. Again, this help can of course be offered
by platonic friends, but sometimes the level of intimacy offered in

romantic relationship can feel like a better fit. I had two partners for about six months during the worst of my health issues. One of them was incredibly attentive to my physical needs, and one of them was not as skilled at supporting me in that way. The former joined me for a ten-day film festival, an activity that can be incredibly hard on my body. Without his love and care, it's unlikely I would have been able to attend.

Different people will also have different abilities, relational skills, and preferences. One partner may have no issues helping you clear your blocked bowels by giving you an enema when you are too sick to do it yourself (true story), while another may not be up for getting that close and personal with your IBS symptoms. One partner might be able to lovingly listen to you vent without trying to fix you, and another might just keep offering solutions when all you need is a kind witness of your suffering. One partner might prefer a date night of movies and snacks in bed (great for a flare-up), and another might prefer being off-grid for a date in sleeping bags (not so great for a flare-up). This isn't just about chronically ill people, ENM can be great for their partners too.

I am *not* a foodie. Eating out is not generally much fun due to all my restrictions and the potential for a bad reaction to restaurant food. If I'm in a relationship with someone who orgasms at the thought of a meal at the French Laundry, I damn well want them to feel free to have romantic dates at fine dining establishments. Without me. Similarly, while I would truly love to join a partner for weeks in the wilderness with everything I need strapped to my back, my back (and much of the rest of my body) just can't do it. I would not want to deprive my partner of that, if it's what brings them joy and they prefer to do it with a romantic partner.

There's also the question of sex. Sometimes my body isn't up for much of it (as much as my mind might want it). In ENM relationships, my partners have the option to connect with others sexually. People also have so many ways they wish to express sexually. I used to enjoy being fucked as hard as possible, but as my health declined, that was no longer possible all the time. Same thing with liking some pain during sex, such as the sharp crack of a riding crop. That stopped being my kink when my daily pain level crossed a certain threshold. I didn't want any unnecessary pain, no matter how hot it had once been. If I have a partner who enjoys sex with people who like it hard and fast or want to have an ass covered with welts for days, I want them to have what they enjoy. It makes me happy to know they are able to express that part of their sexuality (there are, of course, ways to have rough sex or be sexually submissive that don't involve throwing my back out or riding crops).

Non-monogamous or not, and assuming you want a sexual component to the relationship, if your partner isn't willing to find ways to connect sexually that work for your body's abilities, that is potentially a bright red flag. I had a partner who basically refused to adjust our sex life when I began wanting a gentler and more sensual approach. Needless to say, we stopped having sex and the relationship didn't last, for that among other reasons. Chronic illnesses are not a reason to stay in a relationship in which you are not being treated with love and respect, or you just don't want to be in anymore. That goes for all parties involved. But it's not always that easy.

The most common fear I hear from people who are chronically ill and considering leaving a relationship is that they think they will never find love again due to their illness. I do get it, but if you are in a terrible relationship or one that has come to the dusty end of the road, do you really have much to lose? If for financial (or health insurance) reasons you have a lot to lose, it may be time to start moving toward being fully self-supporting. That can take time. It did for me. I had to weigh out the pros and cons. If you are in an abusive relationship, the financial or insurance loss is probably still worth it. It was for me. It's hard to heal or manage symptoms in a toxic environment. I found it to be nearly impossible. When I was ready to leave, I got a lot of support from friends and family, but I know not everyone has that option.

If you aren't safe where you are and you feel you have no options, please consider looking into public social services. There is help available. Regardless of if the relationship is abusive or is just no longer what you want, staying because you are afraid you'll be alone forever is not a good reason, in my opinion. I am grateful every day that I left, and I know that I deserve to be treated with kindness and love, sick or not. You are a worthy and wonderful human, and so many people out there would love to love you. Our illnesses do not define our lovability.

Leaving a relationship that isn't working, when your body isn't working, takes work. It also takes friends, community, family (chosen and otherwise), and professional support. I had one friend who had me over pretty much every Friday night for home-cooked meals made to meet my many dietary restrictions the first year after the breakup. Other friends delivered soup to my door when my immune system went haywire with common cold. My recovery, spirituality, and creative communities offered safe refuge. My sisters spent untold hours on the phone with me, listening patiently as I processed the challenges of being in the relationship and healing when it ended. I had exceptional paid support too, which I was privileged to be able to access. Therapists and coaches who offered specialized help for my unique struggles before and after the breakup made all the difference. With all that said, the truth is there was way more community and friend support available to me than I allowed for. I'm still learning to receive all the love and care that wants to surround me, but that experience did help me grow in that regard quite a bit.

You deserve support and love in big life transitions, just like I do. If you are moving toward a breakup or are newly single, let yourself receive all the help that you need. If, like me, you find it hard to accept help, just take baby steps. It will get easier as you go. It's taken me a long time to build a community of friends who I feel comfortable asking for help. It hasn't come naturally, because trauma caused hyper-independence, harmful self-sufficiency, and a lack of trust in others. This can change and I am proof of it. I've seen my capacity for closeness and interdependence expand more in the last few years than ever before, with trauma resolution being at the forefront of what made that possible. I let people love me now. As for romantic love, I've kept my (limited, by choice) dating life focused more on light and sexy fun since becoming single a number of years back. I'm only recently starting to consider the possibility of reentering a more consistent and committed relationship.

For the first year of being single after a long-term primary relationship, I binge dated. Once every few months I would have sexual interactions with a few people in the span of a week or so. This could be a combo of friends who are sometimes lovers and people who I met online. Then I would get overstimulated (not in a sexual way, necessarily), my pain level would shoot up, and I'd have a neurodivergent burnout. Then a few months later, I'd go for another round. This was helpful in successfully keeping me from reengaging with my ex, which would have been unfortunate, to say the least. Eventually I was no longer at risk of going back to the old relationship, and this cycle grew tiresome. I gave it up, opting for a celebration of singlehood and celibacy.

Before I let go of my dating binges, I ended up having some educational experiences. One night someone I was having sex with was headed over and I was having a pretty bad interstitial cystitis flare-up, along with some intense fibromyalgia pain in my back and shoulders. I texted them to say I was looking forward to spending time together, but that I wasn't sure how DTF I would be, as I was having a flare-up. When they arrived they were certain that my text was regarding an HSV-2 (genital herpes) flare-up. That was strange as I had already given them my sexual health history (a conversation I have before sex acts that involve any risk), and it doesn't include contracting HSV-2. It's also understandable though. If you don't live with chronic illnesses, a term like *flare-up* might not be one you are accustomed to. After that I was sure to educate my sexual partners on common terms associated with chronic pain and illness.

Side note: When you get your STI testing done, be sure to ask them to run the bloodwork for HSV-1 and 2. If you don't ask, they won't necessarily do it. The medical consensus is that because the virus is so common, there's no need. Personally, I like to have all the information so that I can give potential partners all the information. It wasn't until I got the correct test that I found out that I have the antibodies for HSV-1, the strain that tends to cause cold sores (yes, cold sores are herpes). Although I'm asymptomatic and have never had an outbreak, I now always share this info with anyone I might engage with sexually. For folks with autoimmune issues, HSV outbreaks can be longer and more painful, and in some cases can lead to other complications. So it's important to practice safer sex, which includes full STI testing and, in my opinion, full transparency about the results. If you are diagnosed with HSV, as upsetting as that news may be, it's not the end of your sex life. And it's absolutely and without a doubt *not* a moral failing. Having an STI isn't shameful and does not lessen your worthiness or attractiveness.

During another dating binge, I had three sex dates scheduled over a long weekend. I also had a hemorrhoid that had sent me to urgent care the week prior. I had planned the hook-ups thinking that surely the massive blob of pain coming out of my anus would be gone by then. I'd never had an external hemorrhoid and had no idea just how long they can stick around. I'm not sure why I didn't cancel the dates, because by dates I mean getting together and taking our clothes off. My ass didn't hurt anymore (I definitely would have canceled in that case), but this hemorrhoid was so big that if my pants came off it was very likely to be noticed and possibly mistaken for anal warts caused by HPV. I had already shared my STI status with all my dates and didn't want the hemorrhoid to make them think I had been dishonest. So instead of coming up with a polite excuse and asking for a raincheck, I decided to tell all three of my dates about the hemorrhoid. That's right. In one weekend, I had three separate conversations with people who I was not in serious relationships with about my hemorrhoid. By the third one I wasn't even fazed. These conversations, albeit embarrassing at first, gave me great practice talking openly about how the symptoms of my illnesses can come up in sexual interactions.

All this to say, you can absolutely date while chronically ill. In my experience it takes intentionality, flexibility (not that kind), and a sense of humor. Don't settle for less than what you want or deserve because of the stigma that can exist about being sick. Your life experience is part of what can make you interesting, resilient, compassionate, open-minded, and hilarious. You are a fucking catch, not in spite of your illness but *because* of it.

Probably one of the most important, and challenging, things I've gleaned about dating while sick is to set a time limit on dates no matter how great they might be going. The chemicals of crushing out on someone and the pleasurable energy flowing between you can make it *feel* like you are not at risk of a burnout and flare-up. I start with no more than an hour on a video call and no more than two hours on the first in-person date. Ideally that's more like ninety minutes, but I give myself some wiggle room. Setting a hard out for first in-person dates is always a good idea because if it's not going well, you don't need to explain why you are leaving. It also keeps the conversation and connection from being too much too soon. If it's a good date, there will probably be more.

I let people know right away that I have chronic illnesses. I don't give them my whole medical history, but I share enough so that they can understand who I am and how I live. I do sometimes have to cancel dates because of flare-ups and I let them know that too. I am aware not to spend too much time talking about it because I am so much more interesting than some chronic illnesses. And by disclosing it, I also get to see how they respond. Do they get uncomfortable? Do they ask questions, and if so are the questions appropriate? Do they express compassion, or do they seem to pity me? People tend to give you all the information you need within the first date, if you are paying attention. If someone dates me casually or otherwise, my health is part of the package, and I need to know that they can not only handle that but embrace it. Getting a little uncomfortable around things like illness can be totally normal, but if the person seems to check out or pull away energetically, that's something I take note of.

Another simple thing I find helpful is to stick with coffee or tea rather than a meal for the first few dates. My relationship to food is a whole thing, and I'd rather not deal with that when I'm getting to know someone. If someone is a big foodie I'm totally open to eventually going out to eat, but I always eat before the date so that I'm fed and not tempted to eat something that is going to cause me pain. Because I eat a lot of meat, fish, and vegetables, there is generally always something to eat. Unless they state their acceptance of others eating meat, I don't date proud vegans who identify strongly with that diet (I swipe right on them). This is not because I'm an animal-hating, bacon-gobbling 'Merican carnivore. I wish I could be vegan. I don't date them because my eating meat, which is necessary for me, would likely be hurtful and a turnoff to them. One other date-related thing is that if we are not sitting across from each other, I shift my seat so we are. That way I'm not turning my neck or torso to look at them and risking some major pain later on. Small things like that can make a huge difference for me.

The dating system I devised works pretty well, but I use it a lot less these days. I've fallen in love with being single and focusing on my friendships, community, and cuddling with my dog. I also have a healthy client roster, the blessing of my creative work, and a deep enjoyment of spacious, restful time alone. This means dating has been very low on my list of priorities. I feel lonely sometimes, but I have amazing friends who are only a phone call or text away. It's been important and empowering to get to know myself without being in a romantic relationship. I spent all of my teenage years until my early forties, save one year in my late twenties, either in relationships or dating. It's part of what makes me a good couples coach, but claiming this time for myself will likely lead me to being even better at helping folks navigate love.

This celebration of singlehood and celibacy has also given me a chance to understand who I am and what I want in romantic relationships as a chronically ill, neurodivergent, non-binary, and ethically non-monogamous person. When I entered my last relationship all those things were true, but I hadn't yet accepted or even realized it. It was only after starting that relationship that I was diagnosed with C-PTSD and started intentionally resolving my adverse childhood with specific trauma-resolution modalities. I'm fairly certain that if I would have known what I know now and been who I am today, I wouldn't have ever been in that relationship. Then again, being in that relationship is inextricably linked to what I know now and who I am today. I'm looking forward to discovering what starting a relationship from this place will be like.

I've begun to get the whisper of willingness to go on some dates with the intention of starting a relationship (or relationships). I'm in no rush, but I know it will be nice to see and be seen, know and be known, accept and be accepted, and love and be loved by someone who I like to have orgasms with. It will also be nice to have someone to pick me up after my guts have been thoroughly explored.

DTF

When I was 14, I lived in a big old house in a state park with my mother and stepfather. I had a water jug of vodka in my closet. I cleaned houses and babysat kids. I loved cannabis. I was down to fuck.

When I was 20 I lived with my 40-something boyfriend, and my girlfriend lived in the apartment above us. I drank wine and Belgian beer and felt grown-up. I ran a theater company and acted in plays. I was down to fuck.

When I was 26 I lived alone in a nearly empty one-bedroom in Koreatown in Los Angeles, with a mattress on the floor, paid for by unemployment. I went to gay clubs and got blackout drunk and cheated on my girlfriend who sent me money each month. I was driving drunk on the freeways of LA. I was down to fuck.

When was 27 I lived with a roommate and my two cats in a studio apartment in Echo Park in a building that I managed. I was sober and went to AA meetings every day. I was a scenic painter for commercials, an actor, a babysitter, and a dogwalker. I flushed my stockpile of pills and bottle of Scotch down the toilet. I was celibate, but only so I could focus on recovery and then be down to fuck while sober.

When I was 30 I lived in a studio apartment with my two cats after moving out of my boyfriend's house when we broke up. I meditated for hours a day and drank a lot of tea. I was a nanny, an actor, and a meditation teacher. I had experienced a complete paradigm shift due to spiritual practice a few years before. I had met the man I thought I would marry and have kids with and I was down to fuck (him).

When I was 36 I lived in a condo with sticky dust-coated vertical blinds and ugly beige wall-to-wall carpet with the man I thought I would marry but who didn't know if he wanted to marry me. I was practicing ethical non-monogamy. He was practicing non-monogamy. I meditated less than I had a few years ago but still drank a lot of tea. I was a filmmaker, a meditation teacher, a sexuality coach, and an author. I was very, very sad a lot of the time and very, very sick all the time.

But I still wanted to fuck. Sex acted as a pain reliever and pain forgetter for me. My illnesses (which were yet to be diagnosed) and all the pain had been getting worse by the month. I was released while having sex. The sensations, the sounds, the tastes, the smells. The pleasure. I liked rough sex. I liked some pain. I liked to be slapped in the face and called a little slut. I had threesomes and wrote about them. I had men I could call up just to come over to fuck me while they filmed it on my phone. I wasn't checked out during sex, this was mindful sex, but it helped me check out of the pain in my body and in my heart. Mindful sex is simply being there for it. Feeling, seeing, tasting, and smelling. Bringing mindfulness into sex doesn't have to look like making love, it can be a fast fuck with a stranger. Mindful sex is just about being present with your partners and letting go of a goal or destination so you can enjoy the ride. Being incredibly present during sex made it better than it had ever been, which made it a great escape from the rest of life.

Good sex—honestly, mind-blowing sex—made a relationship that didn't work, work. Sexual adventure and multiple partners made a relationship that didn't work, work. Some of the time. Much of the time non-monogamy made the relationship even less functional, mainly because I had a partner who had a hard time being honest (a nonnegotiable for ENM) and who had a tendency to give me the silent treatment when I came home from dates but swore he wasn't jealous. The intensity of my chronic pain and fatigue was mounting and a crash was looming. Sex lessened my despair about how my body was betraying me. My heart was not happy, but sex helped me forget. My body was not healthy, but sex helped me forget. Sex was supporting some serious denial. And I loved sex. I have always loved sex. I have always been nearly shameless when it comes to sex.

People were trying to *slut-shame* me because of my *body count* long before those absurd terms were being used. It didn't work. I can count on one hand the times when sexual shame surfaced that wasn't based on something nonconsensual that happened *to* me but rather something *I* did. I once invited a guy over to that basement apartment I shared with my dad (who was very often not around) and he said no, so I invited another. Choice number one changed his mind and showed up and choice number two left. I felt a little ashamed, mainly because they knew each other, and it was just uncomfortable. The shame wasn't about the fact that I was thirsty enough to accidentally have two men in my underground living room.

My sexual desire has never been something I've been ashamed about. Even when someone I loved shamed me. I just don't see wanting or having sex as a shameful thing. As long as everyone is consenting and there is no abuse of power going on, I say go at it. I think one of the biggest human tragedies is our patriarchal society's relationship to sex. It's thanks to religion, money, and power (elements of the patriarchy) that we are in this dehumanized state of sexual shame. Something so natural being made a sin is terribly backward to me. Despite all our evolution, we still perpetuate such patriarchal beliefs and actions regarding the beautiful expression of sexuality, which is heartbreaking and rage-making. It seems to me that if we can be well on our way to the singularity, we should also be able to evolve out of our most primitive beliefs and behaviors.

I am grateful to my parents for being so sex positive (a little too sex positive at times) and impressing upon me that sex is a good and healthy thing. I'm also grateful that I wasn't raised religious. As someone who has come to Christian faith late in life, I can safely say, thank God that I had a choice in the matter. As an adult I can choose to engage with church communities that don't spew the violence of purity culture or anti-LGBTQIA+ rhetoric. I'm blessed not to have any religious trauma, and as much as I'm deeply committed to my relationship with Jesus, I will not be burning my tarot cards, claiming my beliefs as the "right" ones, or giving up a fun and adventurous sex life. I really don't think God has an issue with that either. Another factor for my practically shame-free sexuality is that I've experienced a relatively low level of overt sexual abuse or assault. I'm a minority in that way and recognize my privilege. That is not the case for most people with vulvas; it's not the case for many people regardless of their relationship to gender. I didn't grow up with social media or porn at my fingertips either, which I can only imagine cuts down on shame too.

A shameless relationship to sex has allowed me to have a career helping my clients heal and resolve their sexual trauma and shame, and to be of service to people through my writing and films. I see my sexual expression as an asset to others, not something to hide or tame. At times in the last decade or so, however, I did *use* it to hide and tame other parts of myself. The parts that wanted to be seen and loved. The parts that begged me to stop begging for love from someone who could not give it. The parts that could see how sick I was. The parts that could feel how much pain my body was in.

This is not to say that I didn't have a good time. I did. This is not to say that after truly listening to and integrating those parts I stopped being a little slut. I didn't. But I did stop using my love and enjoyment of sex to avoid my needs, my truth, and the reality of my health issues. Part of what made that change possible *was* my health issues. I was forced to slow down in all areas of my life, including my sex life. As I slowed down I felt more, and as I felt more I slowed down more. At that new slow pace, I began to accept and explore what it meant to a highly sexual person who also has chronic illnesses and pain.

One of the first sad realities I had to accept was that I could no longer fuck the way I was accustomed. My arms were too weak and my shoulders too tight and sore to make someone cum nine times in an hour. My body was too fragile to be thrown around a room and fucked senseless. My urinary tract was too inflamed to make passionate penetrative love all night. And receiving anal sex became out of the question. All in all I had to accept that being down to fuck like a porn star was not possible anymore. (A note: *Ethical and consciously made* porn, that the viewers *pay for*, is the only kind anyone should be watching in my opinion.)

I was able to accept these changes and make adjustments to my sex life while in the aforementioned relationship. The adjustments were mainly just a lot less sex, as he wasn't open to finding new ways of connecting sexually. Only after that relationship ended did I get the chance to start exploring how my body wanted to relate sexually as someone with chronic pain and multiple illnesses. It was actually really exciting and felt long overdue. My being someone who loves sex, and who helps others heal and awaken sexually, made this exploration feel like a giant missing puzzle piece. I'm still very much in the early stages of consciously and intentionally going on this journey, but I already feel so much more connected to my sexual self and my sex life.

Masturbation, just like the rest of my sex life, has for the most part been shameless, joyful, and free. Currently it can sometimes cause me a lot of pain in my arms and neck to jerk off as much as I might like, and in ways that I used to. Also I'm not always feeling well enough to exert much energy. So for the first time in my life I've incorporated a vibrator into my solo sex life. It wasn't that I didn't like them before, I just preferred my own hands. I had used them with partners on occasion, but even then, it wasn't my first choice. I generally found toys to get in the way. No shade to the toy lovers out there, and these days I'm way more into some vibrating silicone.

My bendable, soft, matte-pink vibrator allows me to get off when I'm not up for using muscle strength, and it can even come into an Epsom salt bath with me. I still opt for battery-free masturbation often, but having the option to not work so hard is a good thing for me. I also like the extra mindfulness and ritual involved with using my vibrator, which is unique from the ritual involved without it. It's not something I just spontaneously start doing in bed at night, which I might do without a toy. I have to actually feel turned on already to think about using it. Then I need to get it from the drawer and take it out of its little silver drawstring bag. I always use lube with it, which means choosing the brand and type I want to use from my collection.

Some of the *divine feminine* or *conscious sexuality* content I've seen on the internet has some stigma around vibrators. There is this narrative that it's somehow not as spiritual, or less embodied. I find that to be kind of (a lot) ableist. I've never really vibed with those very gendered teachings anyway. Even before I understood that I was non-binary I had no interest in jade eggs, gazing at my own vulva for hours in a mirror (gazing at someone else's vulva for an hour is a different story), or polarity. Okay, there was a *brief* period when I was dipping my toes in the masculine feminine thing. But that was only because I was trying to make someone happy who wanted me to be something I'm not. In any case, for those of us with chronic pain or limited mobility, vibrators can be a wonderful way to experience pleasure alone and with a partner.

Another way that masturbation has changed is that I now use it as pelvic floor therapy too. I use breathing practices, relaxation, specific and targeted manual stimulation, and climax to release those muscles, which can get quite tight and painful for me due to interstitial cystitis and fibromyalgia. This is not very sexual for me but more therapeutic. The only thing that differentiates it from going to a pelvic floor physical therapist is that my clit is involved and I cum. Otherwise it's quite similar! That practice tends to give me a lot of pain relief and can help me sleep when that particular pain is flared up. I broke the Buddhist precept of no sexual activity on a meditation retreat once because I was having such a bad flare-up and needed some relief. I don't really count that as breaking the precept because it was just self-massage. And I'm not Buddhist anyway. I am a big fan of many aspects of the religion and of the Buddha though.

I'm also a big fan of being the recipient of dominant energy during partnered sex. I once was down to be tied up and left there for a few hours. Today my joints would not tolerate that. Same thing with being whipped or spanked excessively. I just can't take it like I used to. However, that doesn't mean I can't enjoy submission. One of the hottest things is for someone to dominate me with their voice and eyes alone. That doesn't require any high impact to my body, and for me it's now the best and most exciting kind of BDSM. This refinement of my personal kinks has opened new sexual experiences that have been a lot of fun.

Another fun thing that is low impact is phone sex. Not video call sex (that's fun too) but good old-fashioned phone sex. There is something so sexy about going back to the days before FaceTime and just being two voices creating fantasies together. In a fantasy my body can do all kinds of things without any pain. I think it would be hot to get an actual landline and go analog. Phone sex hasn't replaced video sex for me though. I had some of the best sex of my life with a man in Italy, who I met online, on a video call. No joke. This happened twice and both times we were in shock. He is just as sexually adventurous as me and we laughed and laughed afterward because it was so incredible. This experience was a direct result of adjusting my sex life to suit my body's needs. I feel like I should say that if you explore video sex with partners who you haven't known long, be sure you trust that they are not recording it. Unless that's your kink and you don't care that the internet is forever. In which case, enjoy the risk shamelessly.

Something that has made penetrative sex more enjoyable for me is that I request that I climax at least once before that happens. My pelvic pain and tension can flare up a lot with penetration. It can feel great while it's happening, but later my bladder and urinary tract will alight with pain. By climaxing before anything bigger than a finger is inside me, the pelvic floor muscles are more relaxed. I'm also more turned on at the anatomical level. Being sexually excited and very wet doesn't mean that I've reached full arousal. Vulvas don't jump to attention the same way penises do. They take their time. Making the request to cum before penetration is an act of advocating for my pleasure, and an opportunity to cultivate more sexual connection and communication with my partner. It's also shows me if my partner is comfortable prioritizing my pleasure and my comfort. If someone can't honor that request, then it's not going to go any further.

Chronic illness and pain have deepened my skills of communicating about sex. I was always pretty good at it, but I've become even more crystal clear in stating my desires and needs. It feels good to have that level of integrity in how I relate to my partner and to myself before, during, and after sex. I'm not perfect and sometimes I'm not as clear or concise as I want to be, but I always catch myself and course-correct when that happens. Good sexual communication means higher levels of consent awareness as well. This heightened clarity, transparency, and respect make sex even more fun.

Sex has always been a lot of fun, but it's never been as playful, free, and full of laughter as it is now. Back when I was fucking the pain away, I had no idea that embracing the pain and accepting my body's limitations would lead to more pleasure and enjoyment, not less. For me, chronic pain and illness have created new avenues of sexual exploration, creativity, and possibility. I've been saying for a bunch of years that sex and sexuality is a fluid and never-ending adventure, but it's nice to get such unmistakable confirmations of that. Being sick and in pain can make us lose sight of just how rich and beautiful sex can be, but through accepting ourselves exactly as we are, we are reminded. I will most certainly be reminded many more times throughout my life.

Now 43, I live in a sweet little in-law cottage with my sweet little dog. I have an exorbitant amount of LaCroix in my fridge and an exorbitant amount of chicken soup in my freezer. I am a trauma-resolution guide, an author, a nude model, and an actor and filmmaker. The USA is a runaway train of racism, bigotry, and misogyny, and even though it's scary, I feel peaceful and joyful most of the time. And sometimes, with a select few people, I'm down to fuck in ways that celebrate the body I have today.

Flare-Ups and Grief

On a slightly cooler than perfect Thursday afternoon, my dog and I drove thirty minutes across town to a gated and practically miniature flower-filled park in a residential neighborhood. I don't always take my tiny scruffy dog on first dates, but if it was a socially acceptable thing to do, I would. In this case, he was requested, as the woman I was meeting had already fallen in love with him on a video call.

It turned out that this park was a no-dogs-allowed kind of place. But as luck would have it, the groundskeeper of the park adored my date's long shiny dark hair, beautiful wide smile, and flirtatious flair (she *was* unmistakably lovely). So he let it slide "this one time."

Crisis averted, she and I sat in the shade of the otherworldly purple bloom of a jacaranda tree, on a thick wool blanket she had brought from the trunk of her Subaru—how lesbianly predictable. She also brought me a bouquet of sunflowers and snacks that accommodated my many food restrictions. Not an easy feat and a sure sign that some-one is actually paying attention. This was off to a good start. I am a fan of snacks, especially the ones that don't make me feel like there's an expanding balloon of pain inside my stomach. She was incredibly thoughtful and that delighted me.

Over bubbly water, grain-free crackers, mild hummus, dried fruit, and coconut-sugar-sweetened chocolate, we effortlessly entered a multidimensional conversation, lasting for nearly three hours. Topics spanned cults, ethical *and* unethical non-monogamy, her broken heart from a recent primary partner retirement, meditation, the good, bad, and ugly of those who had reared us, vaccines, weird dates we'd been on, creative expression, and of course, my dog. This was the sort of conversation one gets absorbed in. Time becomes irrelevant, as does the need to pee. Before you know it, you are running late for whatever is next and your bladder is about to explode. Though if you have interstitial cystitis like me, no matter how engaging the conversation is, you don't ever let your bladder get that full.

Although I was able to peel myself away from the layered dialog to pee and keep from activating the interstitial cystitis, I was not so successful at avoiding some of my other flare-up possibilities. I was so intellectually and spiritually delighted by this woman, I forgot about the looming consequences of sitting on the ground, catching a chill due to not packing enough layers, and forgetting to track the potential for overstimulation burnout. I was smitten and forgot about the fact that my body can be higher maintenance than the average able-bodied human.

At about the two-hour mark, I started to remember the type of body I have. This glorious organism that seems to house my consciousness diverged from the embodied experience of the woman who sat, crisscross-applesauce, with me that day. This body couldn't sit on the ground for over two hours. The remembering came in the form of aches, which are always in the background, deepening and spreading. It became harder to form sentences as the heavy and strangely sharp fog rolled into my brain. I awoke from the spell of our jacaranda-shaded picnic-blanket connection to the flu-like symptoms that still sometimes startle me with their sudden arrival. My head, feverish and contracting. My fingers to wrists and toes to ankles, numb yet still receiving pain signals. And my old friend, fatigue, third wheel that it is, cozying up next to me. It had begun, and it was too late to stop the rising tide of this flare-up.

I began to wrap up our time together. This was not easy to do because we had gone beyond meta, and finding the way back to *this was nice, let's do it again sometime* needed a slow dismount. Letting my date know that I wasn't feeling great, seeing as I'd already shared my health status, would have been an easy way to transition into a fond farewell. I recommend this strategy if one has gone beyond the invisible line of everyday chronic pain into a flare-up. On this particular day, I just didn't feel like using that strategy. Instead, I somewhat clumsily cauterized the loose threads of conversation and made my escape—not without stopping by her trunk to get the bouquet of flowers she had waiting for me.

By the time I arrived home, I had hit the wall. I needed two heating pads, pain meds, various topical ointments, pillows, and rest. I fell asleep still feeling awful and foggier due to the medication and woke up feeling worse. My afternoon at the park would likely require a two-week recovery process. I felt emotionally tender too. My date had been thoughtful and attentive, and I felt sad that a stranger had paid more attention to my needs than I had. She also had a whimsical and free quality about her, which was the opposite of what I felt like when I got home. On top of that, I wanted dating to be fun and sexy. Chronic illness had other plans. Noting all of this brought up waves of grief.

One of the first times I met my grief and didn't turn from it was early in my dedication to spiritual practice. I had been meditating on the activity of self for twenty to thirty minutes a day for about a month. I've come to understand self as an expanding and contracting activity of mental talk, mental image, and emotional sensation. This activity can be mistaken for the whole of what you are because it is very convincing in creating an identity. It is what creates your experience of preference for one thing over another. It creates the idea of gender and age, and all our opinions about both. The activity of self is what creates belief and faith. It also creates a sense of separation and makes it seem like you have a fixed location in space. When you deconstruct the activity of self into three strands of sensory phenomena (mental talk, mental image, and emotional sensation), all these creations start to crumble, and things start to get interesting. You come to realize that the whole of what you are could never be just these transient and impermanent sensations, sounds, and images. You contain multitudes and the multitudes contain you. Separation is, on the absolute level, impossible. This is the beginning of waking up, and for me the process started with panic attacks and a terrible, heavy pain in my chest. Sitting with my then meditation teacher and now dear friend Michael Taft, on the couch after his weekly meditation class, I described the feeling. *Like steel in my chest. Like an iron wall.*

He looked at me, in his penetrating yet gentle way, and said, *That sounds like grief. And it sounds like it's been there for a long, long time.*

Wetness welled up in my eyes and my throat tightened with the truth of what he had said. I hadn't yet learned to cry with ease, so only a few truncated tears made it past my eyelids, but the word *grief* echoed through my body, brand-new and yet deeply familiar. Michael instructed me to spend time every day feeling this emotional sensation. He told me that this ancient sadness would change, as I allowed it to express.

Day by day, I fell into this plate of steel, this slab of iron, this grief. I got to know it intimately. At this point I wasn't exploring the psychological content but rather the somatic experience of grief. I deconstructed the activity of this grieving self, not just in my formal practice but also as I moved around the world. The embodied experience of grief had so many nooks and crannies. Layer upon layer, some weighted and seemingly solid, and some more like a flowing river of Swiss cheese. There were days that felt like dying. My meditation practice was a safety line, reminding me that I only had to live through a moment at a time. *It's like this right now.*

Eventually, I noticed how the sensations were changing and shifting, and that the panic and pain were lessening. I had crossed a threshold, and here on the other side were the beginnings of a relationship with grief. This relationship continues to evolve to this day. Periods of grieving have never lost their surprising newness, and I've learned to greet these times with open arms, ready to be annihilated and born again. The beautiful thing about loss is that it points right to the insight of impermanence, which can be an introduction to emptiness and all that follows. You might consider grief not only as a non-negotiable part of being human, but also as a doorway to awakening.

The suffering that often accompanies grief, it seems to me, is *mostly* optional, and each time there is a release of the separate and suffering self, we are given access to the beautiful mystery of what we are. Grief can invite us into what we have always been, what we are *right now*. Timeless and without fixed location. Empty and full. Perfectly okay, no matter what. Of course, for me it's taken years of practice for this to be readily available. The fierce grace of being chronically ill, and the related grief, have undeniably supported this development.

Growing up, my pain wasn't generally addressed in a meaningful way, and certainly wasn't resolved, and I needed to find methods for relief. The first was to develop a tolerance for it, or perhaps better put, a denial of it. You can get used to anything. This served me when I was young but ultimately contributed to many years of suffering and driving my body to perform under duress, eventually leading to a major health crisis. I suppose this tolerance building is synonymous with learning to be disembodied. Drugs and alcohol helped immensely with this strategy. When I took that first drink at twelve, I truly *needed* it. I self-medicated for physical and emotional pain until I was twenty-seven. I'm grateful that I had that option. Drugs and alcohol saved my life, while they worked. They also brought some much-needed fun into my life, until they didn't. My childhood through my late twenties was focused on survival and denial. There's no time to grieve properly when you are just trying to make it through the next twenty-four hours. Nor is there opportunity to grieve when you stay high all the time.

By the time I was in my thirties, I had accumulated a lot of unresolved grief related to my health. Because I had been in pain for so long, I didn't even know how much pain I was in. I was the walking wounded, but in a long-standing denial that kept me from getting the support or treatment I needed. I am fairly confident that some percentage of the pain I experienced was actually a buildup of grief related to being sick and in pain for most of my life.

The way I see it, when grief is not acknowledged and resolved, it can become like a blooming infection, spreading out and invading the entire system. This can lead to fatigue, pain, depression, anxiety, lack of motivation, propensity for addictive behaviors, sex and relationship issues, and so on. Those of us who live with chronic illness are already experiencing much of this, even without the unprocessed grief. For us, it becomes even more important to learn to grieve our health. While it may be painful (and lead to some flare-ups) in the short term, resolving grief could lessen your symptoms, and will almost certainly change your relationship and mindset related to your symptoms.

My acceptance of being sick, and the limitations it creates, has matured. I've come to realize that grief is a totally reasonable reaction to chronic pain and illness. This has supported me in both working through the backlog of grief and addressing new layers when they arise, rather than years later. Grieving my health has improved my health and my attitude about the ups and downs of this body and mind. I've learned to greet grief with an open heart and mind. I let myself fall in love with grief and have my heart devastated by grief. I let grief express. I dance with grief, my body close and intimate with this inevitable human emotion. Or perhaps more than an emotion. This human birthright. I grieve for my health because I love life and all the adventures it offers, some of which I cannot join. Love and grief exist together. I want to feel the love, so I want to feel the grief.

Some grief will always be with me in some shape or form, and I learn to live with it. For example, I will be grieving my father for the rest of my life. How strange the way a relationship continues after a loved one has been reduced to a cardboard box of ashes and bits of bone. The scroll of love and grief for my father continues to roll out, teaching me to be more human, more alive. Even so, being awake to grief and resolving the suffering associated with it *is* a kind of healing.

I carry the grief of losing my dad like a beautiful breathing memorial inside of my heart. Sometimes that memorial hurts like hell, and sometimes it is the singing of a thousand golden flowers opening to the sun. I've begun to experience something similar with the grief about my health. This may be a lifelong grief; even if I fully recover, many years have been colored by illness. When I allow the grief to express in my heart fully, I know it not only as pain, but also as beauty and love. Grief is not one thing. It is not good or bad. Grief just is. It just is.

Over the years, I've cultivated a multitude of ways in addition to my meditation practice to welcome and process grief: writing, therapy, somatic release, energy work, and many other modalities. As time passes, there is less and less to do about grief. It's become an activity that arises and passes naturally (albeit painfully at times), just as seasons change, or tides go in and out. Once I recognize that a season of grief is in effect, I can let go into it, and with that letting go, reconnect to the vastness of being.

Grief can trigger an embodied emergency response that, when left unresolved, can lead to a hypo-aroused nervous system, a freeze. This state needs more than just meditation, whatever kind I might use. I was quite literally cold all the time, and as the years went on, fatigue and low-level depression expressed the deep freeze I was in. I found that somatic practices are quite effective in thawing that frozen state. Swaddled in a blanket warm from the dryer, rocking like a baby. Body curled in, head covered by arms, cooperating with the nervous system's need to freeze and hide. Dancing, shaking, slowly running in place. Gently holding my own face in my hands, like a loving parent with a small sad child. My body knows what it needs to do to process grief. I let it.

Some of the journey calls for doing, and some calls for *not* doing. Another perspective is that there is no solid and fixed me who is going to *do* grief work. Grief, and all the rest of our human emotions, is no different from nature and, as nature, is part of everything—everything—else, from the most microscopic organism to the largest known celestial body. So grief and the aspects of self that grieve are all part of an infinite expression of all that is, was, or will ever be. In this way, there is nothing to do, other than surrender into the perfection of what I, and my grief, already are: perfect expressions of loving, infinite awareness. Remembering and surrendering is all I must do.

When I grieve a new symptom, diagnosis, or flare-up sparked by an enjoyable date at the park, it starts with waking up to the grief. This has gotten easier and easier, as I'm no longer avoiding or denying my illnesses and the related grief. Usually as soon as the grief shows up, awareness contacts it and a simple thought arises. *I'm grieving.* Many things related to my health that used to invoke grief no longer do. The same way seasoned meditation practitioners no longer find an occasional "busy mind" to be a problem in a meditation session, some grief can just cease to solidify into a challenging emotion or narrative. When grief about my health does take shape, the mindfulness tools have been developed in such a way that they come online automatically as needed. Once a sense of wakefulness of grief is available, a simple release into awareness is all that's needed. I know I make this sound easy, but it's taken many years of dedicated practice to arrive here. And sometimes, on some days, I wrestle with grief. It never submits. I eventually tap out and let grief help me up, looking me in the eyes, saying, *Good game, kid.*

Grief is not linear. Grief doesn't follow a specific timeline or particular set of stages. Grief is one of the most multifaceted and mysterious human experiences I've come across. Grief is alive. Though there isn't exactly an art to grieving, we can develop a capacity for holding grief without suffering, while also awakening more deeply to the love, beauty, and preciousness of what it is to be human.

The second half of my life will no doubt bring many opportunities for grieving. Sudden losses will rock me to my core and put to test everything I think I've mastered or realized. Certainly (unless I go first) I'll experience the heartbreak of loved ones dying, including my little dog who is more than a best friend to me. I let myself feel that loss before it's happened. I practice for my dog's death, just as I practice for mine. I consciously contemplate death as a way to be more alive, to love more deeply, and to clarify what has meaning and purpose for me. This is not morbid or "negative" to me. Befriending death, and the grief that walks at death's side, is saying yes to life and to the beautiful and natural expression of impermanence. Still, the truth of impermanence can be agony at times.

I'd like to offer two possibilities, both of which seem to be true to me. One is that grieving is a normal and healthy response to being sick and in pain. Unresolved grief can lead to many varieties of suffering, and resolving backlogged grief can require intention and skillful effort. Meditation, self-compassion, and psychological exploration and healing are paths to resolution and a harmonious relationship with grief. Living with chronic conditions can be made easier by cultivating a mindful relationship with grief.

The other possibility I'd like to posit is that grief, resolved or unresolved, is a gorgeous and glittering ripple in the endless ocean of what we are. Therefore, it is not a problem. It is not less awake than the most enlightened being. That would denote separation, which seems to me is simply impossible. Seeing the truth of what we are doesn't mean we won't continue to experience grief, or that we should cease addressing it in the ways that work for us. As we awaken more deeply, the emotional and psychological activity of grief will continue to process, and it will feel less and less like something we have to *do*. Grieving will be like breathing. Like dead leaves falling. Like cicadas flying from their discarded shells. Like the eyes of a newborn opening to life outside the womb. Like the expansion and contraction of the Universe.

How lucky are we who get to grieve.

A Mother's Love

When a white woman whose voice changes pitch and tone after moving to a place like Laurel Canyon or Bali, or a wannabe grandmother crone with too many heavy crystals hanging from her neck, or a doctor with painless joints and an iron stomach who just read a positive-thinking-your-pain-away book and is on fire for it asks you, with a condescendingly warm smile,

Do you think maybe you want to be sick?

When this happens, it would be 100 percent acceptable to tell them to kindly shut the fuck up. It may be more appropriate to sweetly smile back, letting them see the sharp of your teeth, and say, *I'll consider that.* Perhaps even more advisable, and potentially vulnerable, you might reply, *I appreciate that you are interested in supporting me, but that question doesn't make me feel supported.* I believe in the power of shocking others with sincerity.

We, the chronically ill and in pain, get endless opportunities to practice patience, compassion, and vulnerability while setting impeccable boundaries. I have been more, and less, successful with this practice. Some of the questions and suggestions that have come my way have made my eyes wet with angry storms. Some have made me laugh out loud, others have inspired fast-moving wings to grow from my ankles and carry me in the opposite direction.

Every so often a question or suggestion is truly helpful or transformative when it comes to living with pain and illness. Usually those golden nuggets come from a fellow spoonie who *isn't* a devotee of the Medical Medium, from someone I am paying good money to skillfully hold space for me, or from a spiritual friend or teacher who can connect with me rather than with their desire to appear heroic and wise. In these cases, confronting questions and heartfelt suggestions can offer soft wide shoulders and new forks in roads that have been dangerously windy and narrow.

I was asked if maybe I wanted to be sick many times over the years. I knew that, *for me*, there was some truth to this, but for many years I preferred not to inquire any deeper than to recount that my mother was best at mothering when I was sick or injured, and that my father let his body rot until he looked like a literal zombie. But eventually there came a day that called me into this inquiry in a way I could not avoid.

✦ ✦ ✦

I am thirty-eight years old. There's beige carpet under my knees. I hate this carpet. Truly despise it. I avoid taking in my experience of this worn wall-to-wall monstrosity daily, lest it remind me of how my life is lacking in beauty and instead rich with full-body pain. I'm in my office, and more recently my bedroom due to romantic unrest, at an altar of sea glass, wishbones, pictures of me as a child, white sage (before I stopped buying it), random coins, trinkets, and pictures of the Buddha, the Tridevi, and Jesus.

I have been humbled—wrecked to be more precise—by chronic pain, illness, a nervous system shot from a lifetime of fight, flight, freeze, fawn, heart-racing anxiety, menacing nightmares, unrelenting suicidal ideation, a classic dark night of the soul, and the crumbling of a long-term relationship that was littered with gaslighting, love bombing, punishment, and the emotional papercuts of dozens of tiny lies. To say I am at rock bottom is to under-exaggerate. I may not believe the thoughts that tell me to off myself, but I've still had to fight them daily in the last year.

Atop the dreaded carpet, I have, as suggested by Jacqueline Woods—a trauma therapist and amazing shaman and healer—taken one small puff of cannabis. While I am over fifteen years sober from alcohol, I've become California sober because of chronic pain, frequent nausea, loss of appetite, and general unwell-being. I don't get high, except every so often by accident. This small dose does not get me high, rather it relaxes my body, soothes my pain, and opens the aperture of my creative mind and spiritual connection just a bit.

I settle in to meditate using a Divine Mother practice that Jacqueline taught me. I am working to understand and resolve the aspects of poor health that are related to my adverse childhood, through what I would have once found to be laughably woo-woo. Desperate times call for desperate measures, and bottoming out can expand and alter one's mind in surprising ways.

I connect to the presence of Divine Mother, though I have been invited to use whatever Divine energy I feel aligned with (Divine Genderless Power, for example). I feel her above me, around me. The nurturing and regenerative fullness of the connection I've cultivated is immediately available.

I sip, as Jacqueline would say, the energy into the top of my head.

Divine Mother, please open, clear, and activate my crown chakra.

I see and feel a beautiful lotus flower, in the style of Alex Grey mixed with Georgia O'Keeffe, blossoming from the top of my head.

I sip the energy between and above my eyebrows. I stay connected to the source above me.

Divine Mother, please open, clear, and activate my third eye chakra.

The lotus blooms, connecting my eyebrows with radiance, in the manner of Frida Kahlo, and then I continue to my throat.

Divine Mother, please open, clear, and activate my throat chakra.

When I arrive at my heart, there is a block, and the flow of energy cannot pass through. I feel a deep and sorrowful ache. I pause here and call on my many years of vipassana practice. I get curious about the emotional sensations present here. Equanimity is easily won. Spiritual awakening, it seems to me, eventually becomes about remembering and refining. I have remembered and refined the connection to equanimity for a good number of years. It is available to me in the darkest of times. It's not some special magical thing that was bestowed upon me as the result of being "spiritual." It's just repetition, much like learning to play piano or tennis.

Now I shift into an inquiry practice of sorts. Not in the style of Ramana Maharshi, but by asking the feelings what they are connected to from my past. A psychological inquiry, using the content as information, instead of sitting as an infinite and loving awareness or deconstructing the phenomena. I want to take it personally, to solidify into the selves that are needing to be seen and loved. I need to get into the shadowy, ugly, and ashamed places of my psyche.

No mud, no lotus.

With no warning, I am suddenly faced with the repressed fact that I love going to urgent care. I love being wheeled into the hospital and rushed to a room by concerned nurses. I love being connected to IVs and heart monitors. I love having emergency CAT scans and endoscopies. I love when the anesthesiologist explains the process to me and then has me count down into soft darkness. I love when I get to stay the night. I love it more when I get to stay the week. I love eating the terrible food, being helped to the bathroom, and going in and out of consciousness as doctors and specialists stand over me with charts on clipboards. I love pushing the call button.

I already know but have never fully admitted all this to myself or anyone else. It seemed so shameful. So privileged. So counter to my claims of desiring wellness, or rather my complaints of being sick. I couldn't speak my desire for health out loud, I couldn't bear the disappointment of wanting. I learned that wanting was dangerous, made you a likely target for devastating blows to the heart, and sometimes to the face. I would not want what I wanted. I could spiritually bypass wanting like a champ. So while this revelation is new, I have never surrendered to exploration of the territory. Today, I'm ripe for submission, swiftly topped by the truth I have been foolishly attempting to dominate, like a brat.

+ + +

I am six years old and I'm watching my mother's bottle of Oil of Olay slowly fly around the room. I'm hoping it doesn't fall and shatter because I know how expensive it is, and we had to get food at the church again this month.

I'm feeling a little scared now because the big thick wood-framed windows are opening and closing by themselves, like in a haunted house. I go outside for a walk to the playground half a block away. I've been missing my friends because I've been in bed for days. Looking up, I see there is a big leather western horse saddle hanging in the tree by the sliding board. It's like one of those puzzles in Highlights magazine. Which one doesn't belong in this picture? I know that a saddle shouldn't be here. It should be at the horse farm where my grandmother takes me for riding lessons and where I play in the bales of hay and pretend it's a castle. I don't understand that I'm hallucinating due to fever.

My little kid mind, full of questions. Why is that saddle in the tree? Why am I so hot and dizzy? Why is it hard to breathe? Why do I feel bad so much of the time?

✦ ✦ ✦

This wasn't the first or last time I would ask that final question. I felt bad much of the time. I feel bad much of the time.

A few days after the flying lotion, self-opening windows, and very misplaced saddle, my mother took me to see Dr. Gibbons. I loved Dr. Gibbons. She was big, soft, and square shaped in a friendly way, and had boxes of prizes you could choose from after your appointment. There was a special box that was only for kids who got a shot or something equally upsetting. I can only imagine that some part of my six-year-old fever-boiled brain wondered what a kid could get for seeing a saddle in a tree.

Of course, science tells us that memory is not to be depended on, even when it's not something that happened almost forty years ago while sick enough to be hallucinating. Nonetheless, I'll never forget the look on Dr. Gibbons's face when she took my temperature. 106. Based on the hallucinations, I imagine I'd been running that high on and off for at least a few days. We didn't have a thermometer at home. Her expression was clear, even to a child. This was deadly serious. If a six-year-old can be sobered and calmed with the possibility of death, I was. There have been more than a few times since that I've felt the sobering calm of impermanence revealing itself in this way.

I was rushed to the emergency room, admitted immediately, and put inside an ice tent where I stayed for three days. I remained in the hospital for about a week, slowly recovering from double pneumonia, both my lungs full of thick green and yellow mucus. I had IVs pumping fluids and antibiotics into my veins to keep the fever down to kill the infection.

My veins have seen many more IVs and blood draws since then. Too many to count. When I get my frequent labs done, the phlebotomist and I laugh about my *good vein* on the left arm and how we can only use it every other draw, lest it become faulty due to scar tissue. If I may, perhaps this can be a bit of advice. Find a way to laugh at even the most disturbing of things. Being chronically ill and slogging through the ups and downs of trauma resolution can get quite dark and narrow. Humor is a fantastic antidote to despair and can create expansiveness, even when your world feels small.

If my suggesting bringing humor into your situation makes you want to throw this book across the room, I hear you. But if you're open to it, here's something you can try right now: If you are experiencing pain (including fatigue, anxiety, and depression), instead of saying *I'm in so much pain today*, say *I'm in so much banana pudding today*. Mildly funny, maybe? At the very least, your irritation with the suggestion may momentarily distract you from the pain.

Tricks like that were surprisingly helpful for me when I came to terms with just how sick and in pain I was and had been for so long. My memories of pain and illness track back earlier than the double pneumonia, but it wasn't until I was in my late thirties that I was ready to become consciously intimate with it. There came a day when my physical and mental health had brought me to my knees so many times that there was no getting up and pushing through. I couldn't pretend that I wasn't sick. I couldn't pretend that I wasn't in pain. I couldn't pretend that I didn't want to die. I was all out of the make-believe fuel that had been with me since I was so much smaller than I am now. Dumb tricks like the banana pudding one gave me just enough strength to get off my scabbed and bloody knees and sink into bed instead, letting go of the desire for death and softening around the suffering. A small reprieve into a bit of playfulness was a piece of the still-growing puzzle that has given me the well-being and deep and lustful desire for life that I now enjoy.

My world was quite small, inside that plastic tent filled with ice (especially for a kid with bullying-induced claustrophobia), but my mother, who often slept on the couch by the window in my hospital room, and the hospital staff found ways to bring a little playfulness into my days. A cart was rolled into my room every so often, full of slightly scratchy stuffed animals, bright plastic toys, and coloring books that put Dr. Gibbons's reward boxes to shame. Nurses with tender smiles spoke in pastel matte tones and used kind hands to change IVs, give me sponge baths, and help alleviate the pain (and eventually the seemingly endless mucus).

There was one *not so nice* nurse who was hell-bent on taking my temperature anally. I was not down with the cold glass (with mercury in it at the time!) probing my anus. It wasn't a method that I accepted at home, so I sure wasn't going to let some stranger, authority of a nurse's uniform notwithstanding, violate me in that way. At a young age I was a strong advocate for my bodily autonomy, except when I was robbed of my choice by unkind hands that were too big and fast to escape, or when coerced and cornered. Even the tough as nails, beautifully feral, and wildly sovereign kid that I was had to admit defeat in the face of certain bodily violations.

All the other nurses had been told that I didn't consent to the use of rectal thermometers, and they respectfully took my temperature orally multiple times a day. The nurse in question, in my imaginative memory, looked like a straight-up villain. Tightly pursed mean mouth, sharp pointy features, and glaring or rolling eyes. My mother had to stop her multiple times from having her way with me. I understand that it is the most accurate method, but why this obsession with my tiny butthole, nurse?

She finally got me one day when my mother wasn't there. My memory of that moment is from the perspective of floating above and in front of my body. Akin to how the flying Oil of Olay bottle would have viewed me. I could see how frightened and ashamed I was, half of my face smashed into the sheet, one wide antlerless deer eye in the headlights staring at nothing. Dissociation had become a needed coping strategy for me by that age.

I'd like to believe that memory serves me and that the nurse also felt hot shame for what she had done. I don't remember seeing her again. I don't remember if anyone reprimanded her. I think my mother, in her own semipermanent dissociation, was too overwhelmed by her experience of my experience to do much if I told her. Did I tell her? Was she refuge for me then, a soft place to lay down my troubles, a love to trust? It's likely that I hadn't yet learned she was not a consistently safe container to fill with my tears, while held with love, unconditionally.

It's coming from inside the house.

But regardless of her ability to advocate for me or not, my mother was there. She sat by my bed, even with two smaller kids at home. She stroked my burning forehead, helped me slurp the beef broth, told me stories, made me feel like somebody's kid. She mothered me. And here a neural pathway was formed.

If I am sick enough, I will consistently receive a mother's love. I will matter. I will deserve to exist.

As I remember, it could not be simply a flu or a broken bone. There must be an emergency and ideally a hospital stay. Then I could receive what I most longed for and needed. This message would be repeated again and again long into adulthood. The seductively smooth groove deepening in my brain.

The other perk the hospital offered to me at six was a clean and safe environment with consistent routine. Here I could relax knowing that all my needs would be met. My hypervigilance could fall away. I didn't need to be on guard for my mother's level of emotional distress or track how drunk my dad was. There was no screaming or throwing beer cans. No one was gaslighting or love bombing me, or perhaps worse than either of those at that age: no one went hours, or even days, acting like I didn't exist. The adults weren't too lost in their suffering to really see *me*. I was treated like a child, not a punching bag or a confidant. The sparkling floors, regularly changed sheets, fresh gowns, sterile bathroom were a far cry from our constantly cluttered and dirty house. Meals and bedtimes were set, and kept, by the hospital staff. My parents couldn't even do that for themselves.

What does a child need to thrive? It seems to me that the consistent care I received from the hospital and the love that was unconditionally offered by my mother during those hospital stays were all I really needed. Consistency and love, the best recipe for a good childhood, and a healthy entrance into adulthood, if you ask me. This is not to say any parent does this perfectly, or that I got none of that from my parents; I just didn't get enough, not by a long shot. By the time they put a plastic bracelet around my tiny pale wrist and delivered me into my ice bed, I was starving for the nutrients of love and consistency. Thus, a belief formed.

To get love and care, I must be gravely ill.

+ + +

Again, I am thirty-eight. I am reliving the relief of that first hospital stay. I feel the relaxation and happiness that I must have felt at six years old. There is a full sense memory arising. I've been transported, with some help from cannabis and meditation, back in time. My adult self comes online and makes sense of what I am experiencing. I can see it all laid out, a map of my desire for health emergencies. The reason I long for IVs and overnight stays. Why comfort and a sense of safety always wrap around me underneath hospital sheets. An explanation for the heartbreak I feel when urgent care sends me home instead of to the ER. I can now see that which has always been here.

Sometimes an insight comes like lightning, but not just a flash with little residue remaining. This type of lightning splits oak trees and scorches the earth. When struck in this way, you are changed irrevocably.

I am changed irrevocably.

I know this marks the beginning of a new way of relating to my illness. I ask little me, smiling from the bed of ice, what she needs to release the belief of worthiness depending on grave illness. The answer is clear and strong.

I need to know that I am deserving of love and care when I am healthy.

Tears, laughter, and deep gratitude spilling in all directions. Dear sweet child. Dear sweet me. You are deserving of love and care, in sickness and in health. This I vow to you.

✛ ✛ ✛

That psychological insight was a turning point for me. From that day forward, every single time I have a craving for an IV or a ride in an ambulance (I loved those too), I breathe, place a hand on my heart, connect with a sense of Divine Mothering, and say:

I am deserving of love and care when I am healthy.

I am deserving of love and care when I am healthy.

I am deserving of love and care when I am healthy.

The practice of this new belief has slowly filled in that old tempting groove in my brain. I no longer crave the smell of the hospital, or the feeling of a thin needle pumping fluids and medicines into my veins. Every so often I'll get a small tinge of that old desire, but now it serves as a signal. It means I'm in need of love and care. And it's available to me. From friends and chosen family. From myself. From the loving awareness that has been with me always, all ways. I am loved and cared for, infinitely.

There is one more thing, which I hesitate to share. I don't wish to come across as someone who believes that a change in mindset is all you need to improve your health. Our chronic conditions are real (as real as anything can be in this strange virtual reality we live inside!), and we need more than just positive thinking to heal. And some of us won't heal, no matter how deeply we explore the spiritual and psychological realms. Some of my conditions will very likely be with me for life and some may get worse.

And my health improved after that day when I knelt on bad carpet at my altar. There's no mistaking it, I had a significant decrease in my symptoms and an increase in my resilience. I have to imagine that wanting to be sick, even on a subtle level, was a roadblock to possible improvement. My unconscious or repressed thoughts do play a big part in how I feel and therefore, what I do. Learning to believe that I am worthy of love when I'm healthy led me to take actions based on that sense of worthiness. Which in turn improved my health and happiness. Was I *cured*? Hell no, I'm in a flare-up right now. But when you live in constant discomfort, any improvement can feel miraculous. The insight and resolution that unfolded because of making the unconscious conscious connected me with my inherent lovability and a kind of unconditional health and well-being.

We all have, as one of my teachers, Rachael Maddox, would say, a natural blueprint of health.

She says in her book *ReBloom: Archetypal Trauma Resolution for Personal & Collective Healing* that this blueprint is "a design for physiological wellness with divine intelligence. An organic wisdom that's untouchable, unbreakable, and infinitely available to you. It's always there, but sometimes it gets buried beneath traumatic imprints or difficulties that strike the body, soul, or lineage."[1]

My blueprint certainly showed up on one of my last few days in the hospital, when I heard a song I liked drifting from the children's ward playroom. I scrambled from my bed, no longer made of ice, and on socked feet slid into the playroom and started dancing and singing along, dragging my IV cart along for the ride. I felt such unabashed joy in this free and wild creative expression. Alas, I quickly became wobbly on feet as my blood started running up the IV line attached to my arm, which I had been gleefully waving above my head. Nurses came running and ushered me back to bed.

For that short instant of playful self-expression, I was free from the imprints of my illness and the impossible challenge of making sense of my homelife. I've always been trying to orient toward that kind of joyful freedom. Even my craving for grave illness was just a part of me that was hoping to feel safe and loved enough to be happy. I was silently ashamed of that aspect of myself, setting it outside my conscious mind, exiling it to burn and freeze somewhere deep inside. It was only through kind and curious contact that I came to understand that within my desire for illness was actually a call to wellness.

What if we are brave enough to look at the parts of ourselves we are ashamed of? What if we are gentle enough to let them know it's safe to be seen? What if we are curious enough to ask the right questions? What if we are accepting enough to receive the answers? What if we are open enough to take in new information, or acknowledge old information? What if we are trusting enough to think and act in new ways? What if we have enough faith to know that we are enough?

What if we are enough?

Always and All Ways

My mother wanted to be my mom. She chose me and loved me before I existed in this form. At nineteen years old, she made love to my father in golden Belgian fields and in Grecian seaside towns, every wave of pleasure, a prayer that I would blossom out of their passion. My mother loved me into being. She made late-night promises to herself, hand on her growing belly, that she would never subject me to what she had endured at the hands and fists of her mother. This would be her sacred mission. She would be my protector. I would feel chosen and loved, always and all ways.

But *always* is a long time and *all ways* is an ambitious task. She found herself failing her sacred mission. Soon all she saw was her failure when she looked at me. Then lashed out to try to strike down the evidence, sometimes with words, sometimes with hands. Seeing the harm she caused me meant seeing evidence of her failure again. No matter how she wished it to be different, the cycle continued. I didn't feel protected, chosen, or loved.

I grew angry with hard eyes and a cruel tongue. I once made a doll and a noose, and she found a tiny hanging scene in her bedroom window. Because of her failures, because I was frightened of her and of myself, I would not love her. I chose my dad, no matter how drunken, over her, again and again. The fights would scream between us, an entity of its own. She tried to love me by protecting me from my dad and his DUIs and blackout nights. But her love and protection were not safe or trustworthy for my broken heart. I didn't care what she, or anyone, said. I did as I pleased. I was feral. I was beyond punishment or taming. I was my own frightened and angry protector, and my walls became taller and thicker by the year.

One night, like a snake, I hissed, *I'll go over to his house whenever I like and there's nothing you can do to stop me.* I stormed to my room on the third floor, high on the power her failures had given me. That night was the final failure that left marks on my body and the first that left marks on hers. She had disappeared inside her rage, the same way my dad disappeared into his bottles of beer. The things she did and said are for my therapists and closest friends. I laughed to prove that there was a place inside me that she couldn't reach. I didn't think she could stop, even if she wanted to, and so I fought back. I remember the feeling of my teeth biting her thigh, trying to break the skin. I wanted to taste blood instead of fear and shame. I was all animal fight. No freeze. No flight.

My stepfather, hearing violence, came running up the stairs. He tore us apart, dragged her away, and I was alone. Fifteen minutes later she raced back in and we went for round two. This time I knew to attack. Again she was pulled from the room and I was left alone, my nervous system buzzing. Did I leave that night? Did I hitchhike to my dad's house? Did I ever even tell my dad? I don't remember, but that night forever changed the trajectory of my relationship with my mother. She made some form of apology, but if it was heartfelt, I'll never know. I couldn't see her anymore. All I saw was her failure. I struck down any proof of her love and reveled in any stumble that she made.

Once I became an adult, we both tried to make repairs. I made 12-step amends and practiced seeing *her*, not the things she had said or done. One day, while we talked on the phone, she said something like *I wish I could go back and only say loving things to you when you were a kid*. It was out of the blue and it touched me deeply. I let it touch me deeply. Throughout my late twenties and for all my thirties, there were periods of grace between us, marked every so often by the pain of the past. There have been times when I could pour kindness and love into our relationship, and times when I've needed to pull away in order to heal a freshly revealed layer of childhood trauma. I believe it's the same for her. Our intimacy comes and goes.

My chronic illness inspired a profoundly intimate experience several years back. I had become very ill at a meditation retreat that was on the East Coast, where my mother and some of my family live. When I left the retreat a few days early due to my illness, I went to my mother's house to convalesce before heading back to LA. Before I arrived, my mother asked me to send her the recipe to make chicken broth. She found a place to get the pasture-raised chicken I preferred and had a huge pot of broth ready for me by the time I got there. This act of love and care set the tone for what was to come. I ended up spending about three weeks there, and for the first week I was in rough shape. My family hadn't seen me this sick as an adult because I had moved away when I was in my mid-twenties. They knew I hadn't been doing well for a while, but it's different to see it in person.

At this time, I wasn't just physically sick, I was at the very beginning of a spiritual emergency that was deeply painful, but ultimately powerfully transformative for me. I was also having major relationship issues with my then partner. Between my high level of pain, my inability to eat much other than chicken broth, and my mental state, I was an emotional wreck. I spent days curled in bed crying, inconsolable. I was staying in a room on the third floor, right next to my old room where I had fought back so viciously all those years ago. I was too sick to go up and down the stairs too many times a day, so my family would bring me my broth and tea.

One afternoon my mother came in to check on me and bring me some broth and found me in the fetal position sobbing. I was crying so hard I couldn't talk, and every sob jolted my body, causing me more physical pain. She stood in the doorway for a moment asking me if I was okay and what did I need, but I just kept crying. Then without hesitation she climbed right into bed and wrapped her arms around me. The last time we had been this physically close for this long was in a bed in the room right next door. That closeness left a circular bruise of teeth on my mother's thigh and an unhealable wound in my heart. This closeness is when I felt that wound finally close, not gone but no longer bleeding. I know she was talking to me in soft mothering tones, but I don't remember what she said. I do remember how I felt. I felt protected. I felt chosen and loved, always and in all ways.

My stepfather, hearing sadness, walked fast up the stairs. He stood watching us and offering some supportive words. He was concerned for me, but I can only assume he was also happy to see the loving connection between me and my mother. How long did we stay that way? Did I stop crying? Did I acknowledge the great meaning, and healing, my mother's actions held for me? I don't remember, but that afternoon forever changed the trajectory of my relationship with my mother. I could see her. *My mom.* I embraced this proof of her love and felt compassion for both of us, for how hard it had been to arrive where we were. She took wonderful care of me the whole time I was there, and for the next few visits I made to her house she always had a pot of chicken broth ready for me.

My mother was not given what she needed to thrive as a child, and that has consequences (I should know). She was not taught to regulate her nervous system. She was not offered enough of the love that all children deserve. She didn't have all the therapy modalities we have today. There was no Instagram feed full of ways to resolve your trauma. My mother was actually ahead of her time in so many ways in that regard though. She was seeking trauma healing before there was even mention of C-PTSD in the mental health field. My mother was my first meditation teacher and energy healer. She guided me through visualizations and breathing practices. She taught me to rub my hands together to create a loving energy. We would surround ourselves with that warm glow of love and send it out to help others. She tried so hard, even while married to an alcoholic or in an abusive relationship. Even while she struggled to raise four kids, including angry, feral me.

In the last few years my mother and I haven't been very intimate. The breakup of my long-term romantic relationship shifted what I was available for in my relationship with her. The romantic relationship mirrored what I had experienced as a child, and leaving it made me less tolerant to even a whisper of abuse and neglect. As I've been rediscovering who I am now that I'm free from that partner, I've needed to take space from my mother and some of her behaviors. There are still unhealed wounds for me, and no doubt for her as well. Sometimes healing happens wrapped in a mother's embrace, and sometimes it happens when you give it space to heal without being opened again. Healing and forgiveness are still happening during this less intimate time.

Recently I was in an EMDR session working on a part of myself that feels hopeless and unable to change certain aspects of my behavior and life. Namely poor sleep hygiene and some recurring financial issues. EMDR (eye movement desensitization and processing therapy) helped me connect with how I felt hopeful as a little kid that my parents would change, but eventually lost that hope as things just got worse instead. In doing that work I gained more compassion for the unhealthy patterns I can have with sleep and money. I want very much to protect, choose, and love myself in these ways, but I keep stumbling. Some days I don't do a great job of being my own parent when it comes to setting loving boundaries, and that ends up hurting me. I don't want to hurt myself by not sleeping enough and spending too much, but I've been on a healing journey long enough to know that I can't punish or tame (or shame!) myself into changing. So I just keep doing my best each day, and forgiving myself when I stumble.

The day after this EMDR session I went to an event at my progressive church that was focused on forgiveness. The church leader was talking about the depth of Jesus's love and the extent of his willingness to forgive being expressed through his sacrifice on the cross. I found the speaker's take on this ancient story to be fascinating and emotionally impactful. While I don't think of sin in the same way many Christians do, or think everyone needs to be forgiven of their sins to make it to Heaven (whatever that is), I was still moved in hearing about Jesus bearing the weight of my sins, forgiving me, and dying for me (I actually cried on Good Friday thinking about this). It landed on me in a powerful way and stuck with me as I got in the car and turned on an audiobook I had been listening to for a week or so.

The book was a novel about mother-daughter relationships in three generations of women. The first mother was truly terrifying, though she had also been terrorized. The emotional and physical abuse she inflicted upon her daughter made me feel sick to my stomach. I had experienced nothing like that, though my mother may have. The next mother's behavior was a lot closer to what I had experienced. It was very clear why she was abusive, and how much she tried not to be. She failed at times and then lashed out at her daughter, the reminder of her failure. This would devastate her. Then she judged herself even more harshly and the cycle continued. The protagonist was the last mother and had managed to take a big step in the right direction in her parenting. The book was a decent airport thriller about generational trauma that hit *very* close to home and was somewhat triggering.

As I pulled up to my house that night, something started to take shape in my mind and heart. These three experiences—the EMDR session, the talk about Jesus on the cross, and the novel—were coming together to form an emotional insight of forgiveness and compassion.

For me, the deepest spiritual insights of my life have felt like something I was remembering, not like new information. Of course all is one. Of course there is no self. Of course everything is love. Of course everything is empty. Of course emptiness and form are forever in a dance of love. Whereas the deepest emotional insights usually land as brand-new. They contain information I already had but add a very important additional layer.

I know my great-grandmother had it rough, so my grandmother had it rough, so my mother had it rough, so I had it rough. I know that they all did the best they could and that none of them wanted to harm their children. I know that I am doing the best I can and that I don't want to hurt myself. That EMDR session had given me an even deeper understanding of that aspect of my own psyche. Now this trinity of experiences combined to give me a new insight about my mother.

Just as I try every day, she tried every single day not to hurt me. Just as I do for my inner child. My mother battled her own unresolved trauma so as not to repeat the patterns of her own childhood with me. She didn't fully succeed, but she didn't fully fail either. My mother didn't just *do her best*. She radically shifted from what she had learned a mother was. Just like the mothers in the novel, she must have been devastated every time she fell short of the type of mothering she wanted to offer me. She suffered over causing me suffering, but she kept doing her best each day. She keeps doing her best each day.

This insight filled my heart with a warm loving energy of forgiveness. Sitting in my car in the dark, I laughed and cried as I integrated this new understanding of her love for me. I'd never experienced that level of forgiveness for someone. It was undeniable and unshakable. In that birth of forgiveness for my mother, I felt forgiveness for myself as well. It's so hard to break these patterns of harm. I've come a long, long way, but the work continues, and I deserve to be forgiven for the yet to be healed. We all do. We can all follow our own paths to this forgiveness, religious or otherwise; there is no right way, and I honor and affirm yours.

The story of me and my mother isn't over, and if it were, it wouldn't have a happy ending per se. If she were to be gone tomorrow, there would be things I wished I had said. There are still wounds to heal and love to share. We still struggle to connect, and we may always, but thanks to how hard my mother tried, we are more intimately connected than she and her mother have ever been. I needed to feel more protected, chosen, and loved as a child, and I'd honestly like more of that from her today as well. There were consequences to my development and to my entire life due *in part* to the pain she caused me. But now that is my cross to bear and I do so gladly, with love and forgiveness for her and for myself.

I am open to miracles of all sizes, and a total repair and renewal for my mother would be a big one. Until then, I will stay open to all the small miracles, such as the insight I had that night in the car. Every bit of healing matters. When I am in the depths of resolving a newly exposed layer of trauma and grief, it can feel like dying. When the resolution is complete it can feel like being born again. With each iteration of this healing, crucifixion, and resurrection, I am made stronger and my capacity for compassion, forgiveness, and love expands. In this ever-expanding space of my own goodness, a genderless, dogma-free, and limitless God gently proclaims,

I am your protector. I choose you. I love you. Always and all ways.

Things I Said to Dead Men

I want to write about being ruthless, but instead I scrub the salty chicken grease from a cast-iron pan, a gift from my father that I left in storage in Pennsylvania until he was dead and I wanted to remember him while I roasted meat and fried eggs, and felt guilty and sorry and sad for the time I told him his gifts were the worst, and they often were, but not the cast-iron and not the turquoise necklace that he'd had since '71 and gave me for Christmas a few years before he died.

What I wouldn't give to open another bad gift from him, my fingers covered in newspaper ink.

I want to write about being ruthless, but instead I smear hemorrhoid cream below my eyes and then on my sore and swollen anus, the same brand my mother uses and her father before her, a lineage of trauma making home in our guts, killing my mother's dad one removed inch of intestine at a time but not before I said *you were a wonderful grandfather* and then felt guilty and sorry and sad for speaking in past tense.

I wish I could thank him for being the only adult I knew when I was a kid, my fingers bitten to pink and red.

I want to write about being ruthless, but instead I masturbate and look for the cricket in my tiny house that won't shut the fuck up and watch bad TV because there is too much good TV to choose from and think about the things I said to men I loved who are dead now and wish I could go back and say something else and also save them so they could save me if I stop being able to save myself.

I know I won't stop being able to save myself. I'm ruthless and I know how to dig my fingers into the ground and pick myself back up, bleeding ass or not.

But I want them back anyway.

It's Like This Right Now

Once I had a lover, though he wasn't loving in an obvious way. He was mean to me. I didn't care. I liked the way he smelled of cigarettes crushed between fingers, and motor oil. I liked giving him head in his car. I liked that he didn't try to make me like him. I liked that my years of spiritual practice and emotional healing didn't impress or inspire him. I liked the way we could just be animals together, bodies doing what bodies have known how to do since the dawn of humanity. I liked him because I didn't like myself as much as I do now. I also liked that the hours spent with him could make me forget that my animal body hurt all the time.

The flood of dopamine that came from our usually late-night encounters was a more effective painkiller than the narcotics I was taking every day at the time. Perhaps the numbing of the pills is also what made it possible for me to make a lover of a man whose suffering revealed itself in the sometimes cruel tone of his voice, and the way he hate-fucked me through text message when he was bored. Regardless, I was on board, consensually, for this hard fast ride that gave me a reprieve from the pain-cage of a body that I lived in. I'd say he was getting some kind of reprieve too.

Can transactional sex, such as this, be considered mindful? Yes. While that tryst was short-lived, and I'd sooner never have sex again than have sex with him, I stand behind my opinion on this. During that time, I wrote on the highs and lows of love drugs and, ultimately, through hands-on experience deconstructed my desire until it was nothing more than waves of impermanent phenomena. I took something that was happening under the hood and made it known to my conscious self. That's a big part of what mindfulness is all about. I also enjoyed the hell out of every delightfully debaucherous interaction. I *mindfully enjoyed* it. I was really there for all the sensory experience our anti-lovemaking offered. I made an altar of our unholy union and I worshiped with wakefulness and glee, until the time came for that to cease.

Our relationship (I consider all human interaction to be relationships, regardless of their length, depth, or overall meaning) served as a soothing device for the physical pain I was experiencing, and also as an unlikely spiritual teacher. One night during a text exchange, he was actually being quite kind and expressive in his desire for me, and the novelty of that turned me on. It was impossible for us to meet, and with my warmed thighs squeezing snuggly together, I shared the wild craving I was feeling. How my legs ached, my cunt throbbed, and my mouth was soft and wet. He replied,

Yes. It's like this, right now. Right now, it's like this.

This is a line right out of a Tara Brach or Jack Kornfield book. I had heard it in plenty of guided meditations. Heck, I'd said it many times to students during my meditation classes. But this time, it just hit different. Maybe because of the unlikely messenger. It landed in my body with crisp clarity, reverberating through not just the lust pumping blood to my nether regions, but also into the deep pockets of pain that were sewn from my head to my toes. This simple spiritual prompt made sense in a way it never had before. I was born again, the worship of pleasurable perversity paying off with a new level of equanimity delivered.

Those words—*it's like this right now*—can save a life. Those words saved my life, not when he texted them but later when I stopped being able to have sex because of the pain that would come crashing in and stay for days afterward. Or when my heart shattered and scattered because another medication failed to help reduce my symptoms. Or when I was flirting with a plan for a big crash and splash into annihilation while driving up the coastal cliffs of California. The simple phrase he dropped into our text thread has carried me through the worst of times.

Teachers are everywhere. They are the unkind lovers who we fuck until we like ourselves too much to keep fucking them. They are strangers who love us or hate us on the internet and tell us so. They are the parent who is dead, and the parent who may as well be. They are the kind departure gate agent who tells us to take a deep breath and not to worry, they will get it figured out. They are the friend who doesn't know how to listen, but you love anyway; and the friend who listens to your sometimes unhinged ramblings but loves you anyway. They are the love of your life who married someone else and the people whose hearts you broke, unapologetically. They are everyone you've ever been. The good, the bad, the beautiful, the ugly. We never know when our next great teacher will show up and lay down some truth. Good idea to be teachable, even if you think you are more intelligent or spiritually evolved than the teacher who is offering the lesson.

Did my unloving lover know the gift, the teaching, he was offering me in that text? Perhaps. Under his harsh exterior was a deep and wise heart. I saw it, with my deep and wise heart, even as he tried to hide it with snarls and insults barely disguised as jokes. Regardless, the teaching was received well and has served me well. For us humans who live with chronic conditions, *it's like this right now* could be the mantra, the battle cry, the silent prayer, the life raft thrown into troubled open water. These words are a simple yet powerfully effective doorway into a space of acceptance.

I have yet to find a swifter departure from suffering than acceptance. I let go of the resistance to the challenges of my body, my nervous system, my brain, and all the symptoms that come with those challenges, and I find freedom, even if there is still pain. Acceptance of a migraine doesn't mean the war of pain inside my skull ends, but my emotional and mental reaction to the booming cannons may fall back. The struggling self is what creates a majority of, if not all, the suffering. *It's like this right now* is a clear statement of acceptance, an agreement to cooperate with exactly what is unfolding. Acceptance can help us connect to resilience and peace, even amid the most awful circumstances. Acceptance is also an ingredient for spiritual awakening.

Anthony de Mello, Jesuit priest, psychotherapist, and modern-day mystic, said: *Enlightenment is absolute cooperation with the inevitable.* If something is chronic, it is inevitable. And herein lies a potentially positive perk of chronic pain. Every single time you address your suffering with acceptance, with *it's like this right now* instead of with resistance and denial, you are in radical spiritual practice. Your pain *is* the path. Everything can be a path of awakening, from late-night blowjobs in cars to late-night bouts of acute gastritis. Furthermore, it seems to me that everything *is* awakening. Everything *is* awake. That includes the suffering that slips through the cracks of your cultivated equanimity, or that is simply too wild to tame.

It's all just what it's like right now. And right now. And right now.

Hacking Human Suffering

Pain is inevitable, suffering is optional.

Google can't decide who said this first, so let's just call it ancient wisdom. Yes, there is indeed a difference between pain and suffering. Though often they feel like the same thing, we can learn to separate them and, in doing so, suffer less.

I needed to learn this skill. I had a lifetime of pushing suffering down, which led to all sorts of negative consequences, including many of my health issues. I became much more aware of my backlog of physical and emotional pain when I stopped drinking. Without the anesthetizing power of alcohol, years of suffering came rushing to the surface of my conscious experience. Being introduced to mindfulness meditation gave me a way to move through suffering, instead of trying to escape from it.

Physical pain is an important part of being alive. Without it, we would not have survived as a species. There is a condition called congenital insensitivity to pain, in which a person cannot sense pain. Many people who have this devastating disease die in childhood from injuries and illnesses that are never treated. Simply put, we need pain to live. But for those of us with chronic conditions, our pain can make us want to forfeit life and fall into the hopefully sweet relief of whatever comes next.

The depression, anxiety, anger, and even desire to die that can come with chronic pain are the suffering. Suffering is our emotional and mental reaction to pain. The ache of grief in the heart, the looping negative thoughts, the twisting pangs in the stomach, the resistance to what is. You don't need to have a chronic condition to react in this way. For the most part, aside from those who enjoy consensual pain during sex or *very* firm pressure in a massage, everyone has a strong aversion to pain.

All of this can also be said of emotional pain. While emotional landscapes vary greatly depending on how one's brain is wired, we all have some access to the hills and valleys of emotion. Even those with alexithymia (the inability to identify and describe emotions, or recognize and respond to others' emotions) are not divorced entirely from this human experience of emotions. Of course, alexithymia, while not as dangerous as congenital insensitivity to pain, can make life quite challenging. To experience empathy and connection with others, we need our emotions, the jubilant and the heart-shattering. But when we have mental health difficulties, chronic pain, or just a bad patch of life, emotions can easily become a steaming pile of suffering.

I have found (as have endless others before me) that pain does not necessarily have to equal suffering. It's our reactions that cause the suffering. We repress and resist uncomfortable feelings, leading to more pain, and in doing so, we suffer. When we grasp and cling to pleasurable emotion, we naturally also suffer. *Things are going too well*, we say, *I'm waiting for the other shoe to drop*, and in our fear of something undesired occurring, we miss out on the goodness of what is. We destroy our relationships, careers, and health, chasing pleasant sensations and emotions through addictive behaviors. Suffering of all kinds abounds in this strange ride of life, and us humans, chronic conditions or not, have a knack for it. Hence it being such a big player in religions, creative arts, philosophy, and literature.

My early love of writing and acting was rooted in my suffering. As a young child I expressed creatively that which I couldn't escape. I would likely have a different profession if I hadn't experienced the hardship I did. I also had a deep spiritual connection from very early on. That too was likely due to unrelieved suffering. While my history (and history in general) has shown that suffering can lead to art and spiritual depth, we don't have to suffer to be a good artist or to have a connection with the Divine. I have found that hacking suffering, and suffering much less, has made me a better artist and supported my spiritual growth in ways my agony never could.

Thích Quảng Đức, the monk who self-immolated in 1963 to protest the violent persecution of Buddhists by the Catholic-led South Vietnamese government, was likely one such human. A witness to the act, David Halberstam, wrote this in his book *The Making of a Quagmire*: "As he burned he never moved a muscle, never uttered a sound, his outward composure in sharp contrast to the wailing people around him."[1]

This is an extreme example of suffering being optional. (It's also an example of how deep belief and dedication to a cause, in this case religious freedom and basic human rights, can transcend fear of suffering.) While no one can speak to what was occurring inside the mind of Quảng Đức, my guess is that his physical stillness was accompanied by a silent mind. Of course there was pain, but from the recorded accounts we can assume this man was not suffering, while those around him, not engulfed in flames, were. Their emotional pain caused more suffering for them than he experienced while *literally burning alive*. If it was possible for Quảng Đức to find peace, to be able to light the match and then sit, unmoving, while his body was turned to ash, it stands to reason that most all human suffering can be optional.

It takes many years and intensely dedicated practice to achieve the level of equanimity with suffering that Quảng Đức had. Most of us will never arrive at that place of acceptance with pain. I can say, however, that much of my overt suffering has fallen away through the practice of meditation. The work continues, of course. Life as a human, and this body of mine, continues to deliver new subtle layers of suffering for me to deconstruct and transcend.

The path of freedom from suffering can seem mystical and reserved only for those who have deep spiritual or religious belief. Spirituality has been part of the process for me, but this work of transcending suffering is also somewhat practical and straightforward. An overly used (because it's useful) adage offers a simple instruction for transcendence: *What you resist persists.* Or if you like, suffering is described by my meditation teacher Shinzen Young by way of an equation:

Pain × Resistance = Suffering.

Anxiety attacks are a great example of how this multiplication proves to be true for any chronic condition. You feel the tight chest and fast heartbeat of anxiety, so you try to stop feeling anxious, which makes you more anxious, which makes you try harder not to be anxious, which makes you more anxious, and so on until you are immobilized, terrified, and suffering spectacularly. This suffering is created by resistance, in the form of emotions and thoughts, layered on top of the original anxiety pain.

If I find myself struggling with anxiety, one of the first things I do is soften my resistance and accept the anxious state as it is. This doesn't mean I'm enjoying it. The actual anxiety is far from pleasant, but it's compounded by the struggle against it. Reducing resistance doesn't mean bypassing pain. Ignoring it or practicing toxic positivity is just a sneaky form of resistance, which creates yet another layer stacked atop the prototype. If I hope to lessen my suffering, I must accept my pain.

One of the best ways I've found to cultivate acceptance and hack human suffering is to use mindfulness meditation to separate pain from the reaction to the pain. I learned to do this shortly after I stopped using alcohol to numb and repress my pain. I'm not sure I would have been able to stay sober or find a way to live with chronic pain if I hadn't been introduced to this style of meditation.

This meditation technique does not require a quiet mind, a peaceful environment, a special pillow, or any particular spiritual belief. It does, however, require practice, as does any new skill. This skill can be the difference between a bad pain day and a very, very, bad pain day.

Here is an example of how a fibromyalgia flare-up used to go for me. Let's say it was raining, and my symptoms were increasing, as they tend to in wet weather. My shoulders and neck locked with burning, aching pain. Then there was the reaction to that pain. Words in my mind telling me how bad it is, wondering when I'll feel better, if I'll *ever* feel better. Images showing me all I would miss that week if the pain got worse—that birthday party, days of work, the planned hike with a friend. Emotional sensations of sadness, disappointment, and frustration flooded into my face, chest, and stomach. All of this was in addition to the pain in my neck and shoulders. When these experiences collided, voila: suffering.

In this suffering-reducing meditation practice, you will untangle pain from thoughts and emotional sensations. The goal is to separately sense and accept these threads of phenomena, until they are no longer a knot of agony. As you become more skilled at dividing and accepting this phenomenon, you will find that you suffer less and for shorter periods; shoulder and neck pain, a tight chest, or a racing heart will become considerably more manageable. It's not some sort of magical spiritual experience, it's a skill that anyone can develop over time. Those of us who are suffering every day due to chronic conditions may have both the motivation and the opportunity to excel swiftly. Lucky us!

Here's the practice that has allowed me to hack much of my suffering:

I find a comfortable seat, ideally with an upright spine (standing and lying down also work). I relax my body as much as is available, without judging the parts that won't relax. I know relaxing is an incredibly brave thing to do because it was not safe for me to relax as a kid.

I bring attention to the pain I'm experiencing. After relaxing, it may be even more obvious than it was before, or it may have lessened a bit. I notice the sensation of pain and ask myself, What sort of sensations are present? Does it expand, contract, undulate, or vibrate? What is the temperature of the sensation? How much space does it take up in my body, and what shape is it?

As I explore the sensation of pain, I bring attention to the place where my thoughts arise—my head and around my eyes. I try to let go of the contents and meaning of the thoughts and instead simply observe them: the pitch, pace, and volume of mental sounds. And the colors, shapes, and movements of mental images. I don't try to quiet or shut off the thoughts. I just try to accept them as they are.

Sometimes I also notice an emotional reaction to the pain in my body. Sadness, anger, or frustration might be present in my face, throat, chest, or stomach. I pay attention to how these emotional sensations are different from the originating emotional pain or purely physical pain. The sensations can overlap and be hard to distinguish, but I practice differentiating them.

And then I bring my attention back to the original pain sensations. I deconstruct the sensations into their different qualities. I try to let go of the *concept* of pain and instead feel these sensations, albeit uncomfortable, as simply sensations, and I become a witness to what I am feeling.

When I find myself pulled back into my reactions to the pain or discomfort, I acknowledge them as separate strands of experience. I accept them with curiosity and aim to untangle any knots that start to form.

Even the most painful experiences are not solid or permanent. Thoughts and sensations are constantly changing, in subtle and obvious ways. This too shall pass. Pain shall pass. Pleasure shall pass. This next thought shall pass. All shall eventually pass. I have learned that

I am more than my pain, more than my reaction to my pain. I am an observer. I am a neutral witness. I am the awareness of the phenomenon that is occurring, vast and unconditionally embracing all that passes and arises.

I started this practice with just fifteen minutes a day. When it comes to reducing your propensity for suffering, you will need to commit to a disciplined, formal, daily meditation practice, and five minutes a day won't cut it. You are essentially changing your natural human response to pain, and that takes time and dedication. At times I have practiced several hours a day, which was very helpful in creating this new way of relating to pain.

It was also imperative that I practiced this technique as I moved through the day, not just during my formal meditation. Accepting and dividing thoughts from sensations throughout the day raises your skill level greatly. Frequent microdoses of this technique will increase the benefits and help you remember to divide and accept when you need it most. When the beginnings of an uptick in pain arise, you'll be able to implement this practice *before* you start suffering.

Using this practice, I've been able to successfully navigate away from pain flare-ups and heightened C-PTSD responses. When I first started using it throughout the day, it was very effortful, but over time it has become automatic. It's a new software that has been installed in the hard drive of my consciousness, via hacker mindfulness.

This option—slowly adding the skill of dividing and accepting—is obviously not a quick fix. I am all for quick fixes when they work, but given the magnitude of ways I can suffer, what's paramount is consistency and sustainability in relief. I take a bunch of medications that work quite well, but meditation has been one of the most reliable suffering remedies I've ever found. This practice was passed down to me through my teachers, from the long lineage of teachers before them. Like the quote we began with, this teaching is ancient wisdom, and I doubt that just one human could be credited, certainly not myself or the white men who introduced me to this technique.

An important addition to this exploration of the optional nature of suffering is that all humans are not treated equally. I may have experienced hardships, but they would have been made considerably worse if I were less privileged than I am. There are kinds of suffering that I have never and will never experience, purely because of the color of my skin or the part of the world I was born in. This is not to say that my pain or suffering is not valid, but there are layers of challenge that I clearly do not have to face. I've also had the resources and luxury of time to spend thousands and thousands of hours meditating. We don't all have that.

We *do* all suffer. Every human being suffers. From the most privileged to the least. Ideally our suffering teaches us to have compassion for others, though sadly this is often not the case. I imagine that as more people are dealing with the long-term effects of post-Covid conditions, which can include everything from fatigue and brain fog to anxiety and depression to autoimmune diseases and chronic pain, compassion and understanding will grow for how some of us have been living since long before the pandemic. I met a once healthy and able-bodied woman who has been gravely ill and almost lost her eyesight due to long Covid syndrome. She told me that she felt so bad for thinking her chronically ill friends had been exaggerating their pain and fatigue. Her suffering did indeed lead to more compassion for others.

We don't have to experience great loss and pain, like she did, to consider what it might be like to walk in someone else's shoes. Exploring the nature of suffering through the practice of meditation can help us have more understanding and compassion for ourselves and others. In this way, we can be a bright beacon of love and kindness in this currently ever-darkening world.

For me, surviving the darkness of suffering, my own and the world's, has involved many interventions, including meditation. Spiritual contemplation of the human condition, of my human condition, has lessened my suffering and given it meaning. Suffering with chronic conditions has made it possible for me to help others who are struggling with the same thing. Knowing how dark the night can be calls me to try my best to be a lighthouse for those lost in a sea of seemingly endless pain. Being brought to my knees by despair has shown me that we all deserve a kind hand to help us back to our feet. Our suffering can have meaning for those who are in the trenches. My capacity to love and care for others has expanded, as I've been tenderized by the trials and tribulations of life. When we learn to greet the inevitable pain of being human with loving acceptance, we can heal our wounds and choose what our suffering will become.

Lazy Liar

Struggling to get out of bed one morning, stiff and sore as per usual at that time, I asked my then partner, *Do you wake up every day feeling like you were hit by a car?* His still sleepy eyes took on their sad hue, turning from hazel to gray, as I continued, *I mean is this normal? This is normal, right? Everyone feels like this in the morning, right...?* He assured me that no, it was not normal. That no, he doesn't feel that when he wakes up. He reminded me that I was chronically ill and that's why I woke up in pain, something that I would intentionally forget again and again.

This was a routine we went through every so often, my needing to be reminded that the pain I fell asleep with and woke up to was indeed not the norm. I suppose on some level I thought if everyone felt this way, it couldn't be that bad. I should be able to live a normal life because I was normal. This carousel of pains and infatiguable fatigue was just part of having a human body, and therefore I had no excuse not to pull myself up by my bootstraps and be an able-bodied member of society. But the routine always ended the same way, with the stark reality that my bootstraps had disintegrated long ago and my body was not able in the ways I wished it were.

This intentional forgetting was connected to the denial I had about my health issues. It's a kind of self-gaslighting that I still do a tiny bit now and then. The thoughts go like this: *Maybe I'm not really in pain. Maybe I've been faking it all this time. I just want attention and sympathy. I shouldn't be on any of these medications. I'm just a lazy liar.*

Many years of meditation gives me a lot of space around these thoughts, and I don't tend to believe them or act on them. The thinking occurs as impermanent activity, empty of any real power or meaning. This is possible because I've practiced day after day, year after year, to recognize the activity of the mind and not to take it personally. This can become automatic, but on a bad pain day that has been preceded by several weeks of bad pain days, I have to put in a bit more effort to remember that my thoughts are just ripples in an endless and bankless stream. These thoughts can swim around in my brain, but they eventually smooth out, finding no truth to land on.

A more subtle version of this line of denial thinking comes in the form of comparing my pain and physical limitations to others. I tell myself that it could be so much worse, that I should be grateful I'm not more limited by pain. I use other people's disabilities to minimize my own. This perspective can have a strong pull, and it can keep me from asking for help or accommodations when needed.

During a period when my health was crashing and burning, I also had to fly for work somewhat frequently. Just getting to the airport, waiting in lines, and going through security were enough to trigger and exacerbate an array of painful symptoms. That's before sitting on a plane for hours, and all that entails. By the time I arrived at my destination, I was not well. There was a particularly bad year when I kept going unconscious on planes, once being carried off by a group of paramedics.

Are there people who can't fly at all because of how sick they are? Yes. Are there people who haven't been able to leave their room for years? Yes. Does that discount my experience? Of course not. Yet I refused to ask for a wheelchair at the airport, even though it would allow me to save much-needed energy and avoid the inevitable flare-up from all that time on my feet with my luggage in tow. I felt like it was dishonest to let an airline attendee whiz me through the lines and straight to the gate. I didn't think I was sick enough, in enough pain, to deserve it. If I could walk to the airport bookstore to buy a novel and a bottle of water, I shouldn't need that help. I think there was also a part of me that didn't want to make my invisible illnesses visible, as that would make them more real.

But it got to the point where I had no choice. I could get the wheelchair or not travel. My mother originally suggested it, noticing how long it took me to recover from flying when I came to visit. Although it was a big turning point for me when I finally allowed myself to get the available support, I still struggled with it every time. I felt shame, sure that when I stood up on my two functional legs and walked onto the plane, or went to get that paperback book, everyone at my gate who saw me rolled in would think, *Faker.* I wished I could give a note to each one of them explaining my situation and outlining my diagnoses and symptoms. I found, though, that the discomfort of worrying about what other people (who were likely not thinking about me at all) were thinking was outweighed by the benefit of being in less pain.

I had a friend, who also experienced chronic pain, who I would call from the cab on my way to the airport. I would tell her that I knew getting the wheelchair would have a positive impact on the entire trip, but that I *could* walk. I didn't *need* the wheelchair. Wouldn't I be lying if I asked for that accommodation? She would talk me through why I did need the wheelchair and what the consequences would be of going without the help. I would ultimately agree and promise to text her for accountability when I was being rolled through to my gate.

I believe that one of the reasons I haven't needed that kind of assistance at airports for several years now is because I stopped giving into the minimizing thoughts. I let myself receive the support I needed. By taking care of my body in that way, I wasn't constantly trying to recover, and I could actually build strength and resilience. I needed to accept that I *was* sick enough, *was* in enough pain, before I could start working on improvement.

Part of my acceptance process was giving in to a huge fear I had: being homebound. The fear I had of being sick and stuck at home, combined with the belief that I was possibly just a lazy liar who was detracting from the seriousness of others, more legitimate pain and illness, didn't do me any favors. This double bind just made me sicker. While I never became 100 percent homebound, I did end up at home for a large majority of the time for a few years. I went from constantly on the go with creative work, exercise, odd jobs, multiple romantic relationships, sexual adventures, teaching meditation, social activities, and so much more to being mostly in my condo and saying no to all sorts of things. It wasn't great, but it wasn't nearly as bad as I thought it would be. The surrender to what my body needed gave me peace and a new level of compassion and understanding for others in the same boat. It was also a much more honest way of living. I was so scared of being a liar that I had previously ended up being a liar by way of omission and self-denial.

Up until that point I had kept most of my health issues a secret from most people, or at the least downplayed them dramatically. I didn't want to be seen as sick. I didn't want to miss opportunities because people were worried I would get sick and not be able to show up. I was especially afraid of that when it came to being an actor. I didn't want directors or casting agents to know that my health wasn't stable. I also didn't want people to feel bad for me or see me as weak. I didn't want people to think I was faking it (*you don't look sick*) or, God forbid, give me their endless advice. I didn't want to be known as the sick person. I didn't want to ask for special treatment. I wanted my mostly invisible illnesses to stay invisible. But that meant hiding, becoming invisible myself. I went so far as to do an interview on a podcast about chronic illness during the book tour for *Good Sex* and tell the interviewer that I wasn't comfortable talking about my own health condition. That was one of my many mini wake-up calls. I no longer wanted to live in dishonesty and denial.

When I started coming out about being sick, I was incredibly uncomfortable. I instantly regretted every social media post in which

I mentioned my health. I felt embarrassed after telling a friend about a new symptom. It seemed close to impossible to cancel plans due to a flare-up. Slowly over time, and with my health continuing to decline, it got easier. Friends visited me in bed. I let go of the fear of missing out on acting job (though that fear was not unfounded). I let go of my sexual adventures and found ways to engage with my sexuality that worked for my body. I told the truth on podcasts. I stopped making other people's pain and illness a reason why mine should be ignored. I said yes to the wheelchair in the airport.

Believing my body, accepting my health challenges, and being honest about them has been much like my journey of self-love, trauma resolution, or spiritual awakening. It's not linear but rather a spiral. I remember more than once being sure that I had reached the pinnacle of self-love, but now I know it's a complex and layered journey. After dramatic shifts in trauma resolution, there has been subtle layer inside subtle layer to continue addressing. I laugh when I think about how spiritually evolved I thought I was after having a few peak experiences early in my meditation practice. Loving myself, resolving my C-PTSD, and waking up are not places to arrive at, or trophies to put on a shelf. They are ever-unfolding.

It's the same when it comes to my relationship with being chronically ill. At many times I thought I had reached full acceptance and honesty about my health, only to be humbled by how much more accepting and transparent I could be. This continues to happen. Over recent years, I had a huge improvement in my health, leading up to 50 percent decrease in my daily pain, and the energy and stamina to move back into a fuller more active life. Then through a series of events, some wonderful, some awful, some in my control and some out, I've experienced a major decline. I'm now having to come back to the part of the spiral where I learn to slow down, get honest, and possibly even ask for the wheelchair at the airport. Healing isn't linear.

This decline doesn't mean I've lost all the wisdom and maturity I've gained. I'm learning at a deeper level now, and I have much, much less

resistance to the lessons being offered by my body. Much like someone who had a substance-abuse relapse and then got sober again, I
get to bring what I already know into this round. I'm not doing it perfectly. I don't always want to decline an invitation or opportunity for
the sake of my health, but most of the time I'm willing to do it anyway.
I don't gaslight myself anymore. God knows there are enough medical professionals who will do that for me. This health setback also
empowered me to finally take a psychiatric service dog accommodation. Although I trained my dog to help treat my C-PTSD symptoms,
until recently I hadn't been willing to take the steps to make it official.
I still had a belief that my disability wasn't bad enough. Now I'm done
downplaying my needs and devaluing my lived experience. I honestly
don't give a fuck if someone thinks I'm exaggerating or faking my pain
and illnesses. The combination of being in my mid-forties and all the
humbling experiences I've collected from a lifetime of chronic conditions leaves me with very few fucks left to give.

Not many people would pretend to be sick for most of their life.
Missing out on fun activities, having seriously restricted diets, endur-
ing the side effects of medications, and dealing with the state of our
healthcare system in the US are not things most humans would
choose to do, let alone lie about in order to experience. Even so, it's
not uncommon for those of us with chronic illnesses to question our
own reality for all kinds of reasons. One reason is that this culture isn't
built for the chronically ill or disabled, and we are given the message
that we don't belong. We are often denied what we need to thrive, and
that can lead to us denying our own pain and illness.

That cultural messaging can also tell us that it's our fault we are
sick. I once felt responsible for my illness, and on a deep level I took
it as a personal failing that I couldn't get better. Late-stage-leaning
capitalism and the myth of the American Dream told me that if I just
worked harder I could have it all, including perfect health. Even the
so-called wellness industry and *The Secret* (a movie that says you can

manifest anything with your mind) style of spirituality made me feel like the right supplement, or maybe a coffee enema and some positive thoughts, would cure me. When that didn't work, I figured I must have done something wrong and I should do better, do more.

This fear of being lazy and the sense that one's worthiness is based on their productivity is a universal issue in our culture, as Dr. Devon Price explains in their aptly titled book *Laziness Does Not Exist*. After a mysterious illness forced Price to slow down and *really rest*, they recognized a social epidemic that they came to call the Laziness Lie. This lie centers work and productivity above all and says that we must earn our worth by overcoming our inherent laziness, lest we are seen as immoral. Price suggests that this lie is the origin of what makes us feel like we are not doing enough, pushing us to work ourselves into burnout and illness.[1] That was exactly what I did and, as Price discovered, that is no way to live.

Like Price shares in their book, for me, doing better, and feeling better, meant doing less. It meant giving up and accepting defeat. Through that defeat, I realized I was never to blame, and it wasn't a sign of my unworthiness that I was sick. Trusting and attuning to my body and the signals it was sending released me from both the fear of being sick and of not being sick enough. Being mostly homebound led me to more freedom, and validating my own pain led me to more compassion and a sense of belonging with fellow spoonies. Ultimately, being defeated by my chronic illness gave me a greater understanding of my chronic conditions, including my undiagnosed autism and ADHD, which both had contributed to my health burnout. Having more information on what was going on led to finding the right combinations of medications and interventions, which in turn led to a much better quality of life overall.

I wake up with just my dog these days. He gives me huge amounts of love and soothes any morning C-PTSD symptoms with his cuddles and licks. He also helps keep me on a schedule, even when I feel heavy hearted and don't want to get out of bed. I am rarely in as much pain as I used to be upon waking, but on the mornings when I feel like there should be tire-mark bruising all over my body, I no longer need anyone to confirm that it's not the normal experience for most folks. Living with physical pain is normal for me, and while I'm open to that changing, I can honor the truth and base my choices and actions on that truth. My pain is real. I'm not a lazy liar.

Upon Waking

This morning before the coffee, before the necessary food, before the medications that offer the golden ticket to getting through the day, before I try to move this body, before I hold my own heart and say *I love you*, before I hold the space that helps others do the same, before I wash the residue of hurts they've carried from my hands with salt and water, before I practice having fun, before I let the artist come out to play, before I tell the child with no bedtime and no routine who lives inside me that it's time to sleep, before I stay up later anyway, before I sleep again to do it all again.

+ + +

Before all this there is a moment of remembrance.

+ + +

I remember that I get to be here.

I remember that some strange and miraculous turn of events allowed for me to exist.

I remember that there is no guarantee that I will do it all again tomorrow.

I remember that the love I have felt in this *one wild and precious life* greatly outweighs the pain, no matter what the suffering says when it wakes from its slumber.

+ + +

The suffering sleeps gently most days now.

It visits only in flashes of sensation and thought,

recognized to have meaning, purpose, even value, but not to be the whole of me.

✦ ✦ ✦

More and more it seems that remembering is the essential practice for refining this human that is me.

✦ ✦ ✦

More and more it seems that remembering is the essential practice for awakening to all that is beyond this human that is me.

✦ ✦ ✦

Remember this: You are here and it is now.

Gold Linings

Driving, windows down, dried streaks of salty tears on my cheeks, scream-singing *What doesn't kill you makes you stronger*. The pop song was doing what good pop songs do to me: finding its way past my logical and intellectual mind and into the bloody meat of my heart. I was in a relationship that was not making me feel strong and often felt like *it* would kill me, but I was a ways off from leaving. In my mid-thirties I felt like I had plenty of time to spare, not knowing how fast forty would come. I may have spent less time crying to pop music if I had known. But I didn't, and Clarkson's song, which borrows the oft-quoted words of Nietzsche, registered empowering to my shaky breaky heart and trauma-bond-fogged mind.

At that time I knew much less about how trauma affects the mind and body, so I could get on board with the idea that we can be forged in the fire of abuse and become more powerful and resilient than before. Although this can be true, sometimes it just isn't that simple, especially when one has already had repeated stressors or traumas. A team of researchers from Brown University and the University of Concepción studied 1,160 Chileans before and after the earthquake and tsunami of 2010. Among the 9 percent who developed PTSD and the 14 percent diagnosed with major depressive disorder, their common denominator tended to be a history of stressful or traumatic experiences before the natural disasters hit their country, researchers found.[1] Science points to PTSD leading to health issues, so along with the mental health toll we can imagine there was an effect on physical health as well.[2]

The study of Chilean natural-disaster survivors illustrates what those of us who have spent years resolving trauma know very well. What doesn't kill us can make us more susceptible to mental and physical health issues. For myself, I can also say that my history of trauma seems to have led to psychological patterns in which I re-created and reopened old wounds, making my body and mind even more vulnerable to pain and suffering. So as much as I might enjoy the sentiment in theory (or in catchy girl-power pop music), Nietzsche can, respectfully, kiss my ass.

The idea that we are supposed to overcome all adversity, pull up our bootstraps, get back on the saddle, and come out victorious no matter the circumstances feels like it's pulled right out of the *How to convince people that late-stage capitalism, systemic racism, and the patriarchy are totally cool* handbook. It's already a feat to resolve and recover from our own personal hardships, but we also have our generational and ancestral wounds. On top of that we live in a web of systems that harm us. Even those who benefit from these systems are being harmed by them too. As much as we do to rid ourselves of the weight of our own trials and tribulations, the infection of trauma is still in the water. *Literally*—our oceans are polluted, the ice caps are melting, and drinking water is being poisoned in the name of their god, oil.

A lack of traumatic events still doesn't guarantee a perfect life full of everlasting happiness and bliss. Suffering is part of being human. But living trauma-free sure can make life a lot easier. People who have consistent loving caretakers, grow up untouched by poverty or abuse, receive excellent educations, and are given access to all the resources they need in order to thrive have quite a leg up in the game of life. They are stronger because they have been strengthened. This fortification, which begins while they are still in the womb, sets them up to succeed. I have, in moments of grief or frustration, thought about how much easier life would have been (and would be today) if I had been offered a solid and safe foundation from the beginning. I wonder, *Who would I have been?*

I want to explore the concept of post-traumatic growth without negating the fact that C-PTSD, and much that it comes with, sucks. Being told to look for the silver lining of abuse, neglect, and the inherent trauma of being human in a world that is often so dehumanizing can be one of the least helpful suggestions ever. Especially when it comes from someone who has no clue what it's like to have been in a state of flight, fight, or freeze for most of your life. I know what that's like. I also know that many of the painful and damaging things that have occurred in my life have been lined with silver. In fact, I'd go so far as to say they have been lined with gold.

When I researched the term *gold lining* to see how others were using it, I came across an article by Andrew Carlin called *From Silver to Gold Lining; From Comparative to True Gratitude.*[3] Written during his graduate research fellowship at Duke, Carlin speaks about the difference between comparative gratitude and *true* gratitude. Comparative gratitude (*I should be grateful I was only emotionally abused by my parents, some people are physically abused. It could have been so much worse*) creates the tendency to belittle and invalidate our own traumatic experiences, which means we may not be able to heal from them and grow. He also aptly notes that this sort of gratitude can lead us to stay in unhealthy relationships (*They only call me names and yell at me, I should be grateful I have a partner. It could be so much worse*). This idea inspired me to begin this exploration of the gold lining of trauma with the topic of gratitude.

The theory of post-traumatic growth was developed in the mid-1990s by psychologists Richard Tedeschi, PhD, and Lawrence Calhoun, PhD.[4] Simply put, post-traumatic growth is the positive personal changes and growth that can occur because of trauma. This is different from resilience, the ability to bounce back from difficult experiences, as it's the growth that comes from *not* being able to recover quickly. The type of personal changes based in going to the depths of despair and making it out alive. Think a sparkling diamond, formed in darkness through intense heat and pressure. Or the process of a landbound caterpillar transforming into a majestic butterfly, by first digesting itself and turning to ooze. A diamond doesn't bounce back to being a carbon deposit. A butterfly doesn't recover to become a caterpillar again. They are changed into something else entirely. Something beautiful. The theory of post-traumatic growth says that our traumas can change us in beautiful ways, not in spite of hardships but because of them.

As a reminder, experiencing any of these positive changes *does not mean* that what happened to you was okay, or that your past suffering can be brushed off your shoulders like so much dust. The truth of the trauma you endured is not something you need to be grateful for. I don't dig the sayings *Everything happens for a reason* or *God won't give you anything you can't handle.* Sometimes terrible stuff just happens, and I don't think God (or any higher power) is doling out trauma thinking, *Oh yeah, they can handle that, I think I'll throw another illness or awful breakup on the pile, they've got it!* Also, it's important to mention that not everyone who is carrying trauma experiences post-traumatic growth in the way it's described here, but that doesn't mean that they can't heal and grow in all kinds of ways. This is just one model of what trauma resolution can look like.

The following are the recognized criteria for post-traumatic growth.[5] Although this list was developed based on studies involving PTSD (limited to single or short-duration traumatic events), in my experience, and that of many of my clients, it aligns with the positive changes that can occur through the resolution of complex-PTSD as well.

+ Appreciation of life

  Going through hell, and coming out the other side, can offer a heightened awareness of the precious and transient nature of existence and show you just how beautiful, rich, and complex life can be.

+ Relationships with others

If you've been to hell, you may have greater empathy and understanding for those who are traversing similar terrain, which can increase the chance of deeper emotional connections and meaningful bonds in your relationships.

+ New possibilities in life

After surviving hell, things that once seemed impossible may no longer feel so out of reach, and the wisdom you gained through adversity can translate into an evolved understanding of what holds meaning for you.

+ Personal strength

Climbing out of the depths of hell can build some powerful mental and emotional muscles, leading to the strength and resilience to weather just about any storm life throws your way.

+ Spiritual change

The suffering that hell brings, as well as release from that suffering, can inspire profound spiritual insights regarding the nature of reality, such as the interconnection of all things or universal love, and may deepen your sense of faith and trust in personal intuitive wisdom or a higher power. It has been true for me that appreciation of life has increased as a result of trauma, and I believe that gratitude is part of what brought me to the other side from an incredibly dark and traumatic period of my life.

Shortly after my first book came out, I went to a monthlong silent retreat in the woods of Massachusetts at a center for seasoned meditation practitioners. It was self-led, and other than a fifteen-minute check-in session twice a week with a resident teacher, I was on my own. I saw people in the meditation hall, but most of us meditated in our private rooms. There was also mealtime, but my health quickly crashed after a week of eating the delicious food that was not part of my restriction-heavy diet, and I had to switch to a simple-foods diet that I made for myself. So meals were also basically solo. Even if that wasn't the case, the meals were not a time to be social, as it was a *silent* retreat center.

I got quite sick on the retreat and ended up in the hospital. In all honesty I had no business going on that retreat, due to my health limitations, but I just really wanted to give it a try. I left the retreat at twenty-eight days instead of the planned thirty-five and headed to my mother's house in Pennsylvania to convalesce. Then all hell broke loose. I couldn't stop crying, but I also felt numb and hollow. I was flooded with thoughts of suicide and could find little meaning in life. There was a series of fractures and betrayals in my romantic relationship that I couldn't suffocate with denial. The constant physical pain I was experiencing had hit an all-time high. I was miserable but couldn't break through the endless sea of apathy I was drowning in to do much to help myself.

What I didn't know until a year of hell later was that I had entered a classic Dark Night of the Soul, a term coined by Saint John of the Cross, a Catholic mystic and poet. This is a period of total spiritual desolation, devastation, and depression. You can feel completely disconnected from faith in your spiritual path or religious beliefs. There can be a sense that you have lost all access to being a somebody and are unable to find a way back to yourself. All solid ground seems to crumble, and you fall into terrifyingly meaningless and empty existence. The dark night of the soul is a true spiritual emergency. This is not just a *hard time*; this is, as my teacher Shinzen Young says, *the pit of the void*. This can be a side effect of meditation, which is why I very openly talk about the dark side of meditation. It's not all less stress, better sex, more compassion. Some types of meditation, especially when paired with trauma, can also wreak havoc on your mental health and over all well-being. Highly intense side effects are not incredibly common, but I believe in informed consent and think that it's important to be aware of.

For me, dark night felt like my plug had been pulled and I was emptied out—and not in a good way. It wasn't just a bit of existential angst and feelings of meaninglessness, I felt as if I was being dragged into a black void of annihilation. In addition to some primal layers of trauma that had surfaced in the isolation of the retreat, the extreme of a month of meditation launched me into this spiritual emergency. Part of what I experienced was suicidal ideation, daily for eight months. It was soul draining.

The tricky thing with dark night is that it will feast on any material you offer it. A major component of my experience was intrusive rumination, and for the first five months of this time of darkness, I kept getting pulled into stories related to the issues in my life. My primary romantic relationship was in shambles, and I was obsessed with all the ways I had been mistreated or betrayed and how to fix the unfixable. I was broke and in debt and was sure I'd never be able to find my way out of the financial quagmire. My health was declining rapidly, and I had lost all hope that I would ever improve. I was caught in loops of suffering about my woes. Because I had been meditating for a long-ass time, I could very easily see through the suffering, but it was relentless nonetheless. At the time a friend described the state as *when you know there is no cage, but you are still in the cage.* Indeed. At a certain point, I stopped feeding the demon, my anxious thoughts about health, money, and love. Then it was just the black void. This was when I stopped trying to fix the things my mind was telling me were the issue, and started addressing the depth of despair and disillusionment I was adrift in.

Desperate for relief, I turned to Dr. Joe Dispenza, mind-body spiritual teacher. For the record, I find some of his stuff very *The Secret*-y and coming from an assumption of privilege. Nonetheless, I find some of his work to be highly effective and helpful. There is a forty-five-minute practice on letting go of negative beliefs and cultivating new ones that I stumbled across one day. I used his guidance to an extent, but also went off-roading quite a bit. In my opinion, we are all our own best teacher. It's important to trust our own inner compass, as well as follow the guidance of a teacher.

In the practice, Dispenza guides you into an endlessly vast and spacious *no self* state. Then you bring up the belief you want to let go of and release it into the ether. My unwanted belief was that life was over, there would never be joy again, and I should die. Once you release the negative belief, Dispenza guides you in bringing up a positive new belief. At that time, I didn't dare try to cultivate joy, that seemed much too far away. Instead I focused on peace and safety. The instruction is to use your imagination to see it as already true, and then to feel in your body that truth. I had a series of fantasies related to peace and safety that, when played out in my mind, would vibrate through my body. I was essentially practicing feeling what I wanted to feel. Toward the end of the practice, he guides you to a place of gratitude for receiving what you want, even before it has happened. This boost of gratitude seems to supercharge the power of my imagination, making the feelings even more real.

I used this practice day after day (in conjunction with breathwork, ice-cold showers, EMDR therapy, and other modalities and guidance), and I did slowly start to feel safer and more peaceful. I also felt immense gratitude for the few things that seemed to break through the darkness. Mainly my niece's and nephews' FaceTime calls. I nurtured that gratitude as much as I could, as well as any bit of gratitude for simple things like sun on my back or the purr of my cat. Where before I was stuck in intrusive rumination, I was now using deliberate rumination to cultivate gratitude.

Although it was some time before I was out of the midnight forest of misery, I can attest that all the gratitude started to make a difference.

One afternoon I was kneeling on the beige carpet of my condo, praying for relief, and I heard myself say *I don't care what my job is, where I live, what my financial situation is, or how bad my health is, I just want to experience some amount of peace and happiness. I am so grateful for anything that offers me that.* I realized that none of what I thought mattered actually mattered at all. There had been plenty of insight about this in my many years of spiritual practice, but this went soul-deep and irrevocably changed me.

I was still having daily thoughts of suicide and had even started to consider how I might do it, but not long after this moment on my knees, I decided to stop allowing those thoughts. I wanted gratitude to take the wheel instead. I had my last unaliving daydream hurrah before a solo trip up the California coast. I let myself imagine smashing on the rocks at the bottom of the cliffs, and then I said, *No more.*

From there on out, if even a whisper of one of those thoughts came up, I extinguished it like a kitchen fire. Fast and with no hesitation. I would often redirect to something I was grateful for. These would be small everyday gratitudes. After about five months of negating those thoughts, for one instance I let suicidal ideation burn. I gave myself two minutes, and it was such a relief. I wasn't in total crisis anymore, and I did feel peaceful and relatively safe, but the dark void hadn't gone, and it still called me to oblivion.

Around that time, I reached out to Shinzen Young and told him what was going on. Why I hadn't reached out sooner during that time of darkness I cannot say. I certainly would have saved myself some anguish. On that call I said I thought I had some sort of serious depression, but that it didn't seem like any depression I had ever known. In his great wisdom, he asked me several questions, told me that I was experiencing a dark night of the soul, and gave me the simple instructions to notice the connectivity and fulfillment within everything, including the pit of the void. Between that, some trauma resolution for my infant and in utero self, and a few powerful shamanic practices, I was feeling a lot better within a month and back in the bright light of dawn within about four months. It took another few years before I discovered a new joy that would replace what I once experienced as joy, but I no longer felt the call of death, and I was able to find enjoyment in life again.

It's taken years for me to fully integrate and understand what I experienced during that time. It was incredibly traumatic and was enlaced with my C-PTSD. It also changed my life for the better in so many ways. I wish it hadn't had been so hard on me and on my loved ones, who could do very little to help as I suffered, and I'm full of gratitude for what I learned and how I grew as a result. After going to that level of despair, I also appreciate life in a way that I never did before. Gratitude helped me gain freedom from the intrusive rumination, and more gratitude, aka appreciation of life, showed up because of post-traumatic growth. It's important to note that the comparative gratitude didn't work for me—I needed the *true* gratitude that Andrew Carlin wrote of. Being grateful based on how much more I perceived someone else to be suffering only created a sense of shame and repressed the pain I was in. True gratitude and deliberate positive rumination are what allowed me to move out of the suicidal ideation.

I now think of the rumination on suicide in a very different way. I see it now as a call to connection and fulfillment with the Divine. Before I understood what I was experiencing, I could only sense the draw to annihilation as a desire to die. I didn't realize that I could be regenerated by the emptiness, be reborn again and again into the beauty and fullness of life. Today when I get whispers of a desire to die, I automatically remember that physical death is not necessary to be held by the loving embrace of God (I resonate with that word, but you don't need to believe in any sort of higher power to experience unity, love, and fulfillment in this way).

Within this story, there are examples of the other four criteria for post-traumatic growth. My relationships with others deepened exponentially through this experience. I grew closer to my siblings, I had some very healing moments with my mother and stepfather, and the friends who stuck around are now my ride-or-die humans. I also came to understand the struggles of my loved ones, my clients, and humans in general in a much more personal way. This increased the intimacy and connection that was possible in all my relationships, including that with humanity at large. I also started a new relationship with a tiny and adorable scruffy dog named Jake Billie Twist. He is one of the best things to ever happen to me, and I don't think I would have allowed myself to invite him into my heart if it hadn't been for the expansion in my capacity for intimate relationships.

This traumatic time also ushered in new possibilities in life. Because I was unable to do much else, I grew my business. Within a few years I had doubled my income and had a roster of wonderful clients. It's interesting to think that during the darkest time, I was able to be a light for others. That was partially because of all the new access to compassion I had, and partly because there was lot less *me* to get in the way of an intuitive connection with my clients and with what they needed. I also came to understand that I wanted to support others with spiritual emergency and the side effects of meditation, and made that a cornerstone of my offerings. In addition I realized that I had a great passion for trauma resolution and wanted to focus on that in my work with clients. I have since become certified in somatic trauma resolution and archetypal post-traumatic growth guidance and have been trained to offer brainspotting, a powerful modality that is an off-shoot of EMDR.

As for personal strength and spiritual change, that time of my life most certainly resulted in both of those. I eventually had the strength to leave the relationship that was harmful for me. That required major upheaval, but I had gained so much resilience through the process of moving from darkness to light that I wasn't afraid. I also became strong enough to overcome the addictive patterns I had been playing out in that relationship. There was strength required to come out as non-binary and to address my neurodivergence, and I gained some of that strength by going to hell and back. Perhaps where I have really seen the post-traumatic growth express through personal strength is how much more comfortable I am with vulnerability. I was forced to learn to ask for help and to allow others to love and support me. I now let my loved ones see my pain and my joy. I let them see *me.*

I had a big awakening experience in my first year of serious meditation practice, akin to being unplugged from the Matrix. The massive paradigm shift was unmistakable and life changing. Following that were years of practice, deepening of insight, and tons of trauma recovery, which is 100 percent necessary for anyone on a spiritual path who has experienced trauma. Meditation isn't a silver bullet. Eventually, after a stabilization of all that had occurred in my practice, I was given the instruction by Shinzen to simply focus on refining the human. It wasn't long after that when I fell into the pit of the void. Then two years later at a retreat led by Shinzen, over a decade after that first reality-shattering awakening, all the insights that had arisen as a result of my practice converged. The infinite dance of emptiness and form, once an occasional reality, was revealed as the unconditional home that had always been there. A spontaneous and joyful peace became consistently and easily available, even in moments of heartbreak and pain. Since that retreat, there has been a mostly uninterrupted trust and faith in the flow of life. *Everything* feels easy most of the time, and even when challenge arises, there is an inextinguishable and unconditional happiness holding it all.

The year I spent navigating the depths of darkness was also a time of addressing aspects of C-PTSD that I had never previously touched, and the constant low-level trauma of being in a relationship that kept reopening my core traumas from childhood. That work continued and the post-traumatic growth I experienced grew as I resolved more and more of that material. To this day, I am delighted by how post-traumatic growth keeps showing up in my life. Most recently, because of addressing some sleep and financial issues related to C-PTSD, I've entered an entirely new way of engaging with my spiritual life. I've found a level of love and care from God that I never allowed myself to receive before now. This new access to Divine support has been opening so many doors for me, in all realms of life. There may not be much science on it yet, but I feel confident that in the not-too-distant future there will be strong evidence to support the presence of post-traumatic growth for those of us not just with PTSD but also those with C-PTSD.

We began with a quote from Nietzsche that, while it holds a level of truth, seems to lack the miraculous and graceful beauty that I associate with post-traumatic growth. Let us end with this eloquent line from the essay "Return to Tipasa" by Albert Camus: "In the midst of winter, I found there was, within me, an invincible summer."[6]

That invincible summer is inside all of us, no matter how long and cold the winter has been. The sun is shining and skies are clear. There is glorious and wild space to roam, and soft and safe places to rest. Here you are enough, as you always have been, and always will be.

May you find the gold linings, wherever they appear.

ACKNOWLEDGMENTS

I must express endless gratitude to the skilled and compassionate trauma practitioners who have been part of my C-PTSD resolution journey: Rachael Maddox, Christine Ashe, Lee Ann Teaney, Barbara Herring, Ezrimayr Chioma, and Jacqueline Woods. A massive thank-you to Kendall Haydel and Crystal I. Lee for the life-changing diagnoses of ADHD and autism.

I'm also incredibly thankful to the other members of my support team on the recent leg of my journey of healing and awakening: Shinzen Young, Dr. Soha Dolatabadi, Michael Taft, Jackie Shea, Gena Ferrabee, Brett Fleisher, Christine Rose Elle, Britt Sulkin, Tracy McMillan, Raina DeLear, Ed, Hannah, Raul, Nelly, and the Bread Community, Pastor Jes and the LA church community, Judy Esber, and Gail Bradley.

Thank you to Shayna Keyles, Bevin Donahue, Margeaux Weston, Tim McKee, and the team at North Atlantic Books. It means the world to me that you championed me in taking this next step in my creative work.

Many thanks to Stef Estep-Gozalo and Christine Little for being sensitivity readers. Thank you to Tyler Johnson for coming to the rescue with some last-minute help during the early stages of this book. I'm so grateful to my dear friend Shayan Asgharnia for another phenomenal author portrait and for being one of the few humans in LA who I wanted babysitting me after I was under anesthesia. A massive thank-you to Maria Olson for her consistent love, support, and guidance with the completion of this book and as a sister-friend and imaginary podcast co-host.

There are so many loved ones who have helped me be the person who could write this book, along with helping me in a bunch of other ways in recent years. Thank you to my sisters Dian and Melanie, my brother Sam, Sharon Sim, Mia Siracusa, Dani De Luca, Martha Propser, Whitney Ullom, Robert Dowdy, Lauren Maher, Dustin Ingram, Jeff Kober, Adele Slaughter, Tamara Levitt, Jenn Howd, Shauna Shapiro, Deb Fisher, Kashi Ananda, Doug Hurley, Alex P. Gutterman, Rachel Brookner, Walker Davis, Jordan Lane Shappell, Mike Hackett, Joshua Bitton, Sochi Thomas, Elsa Nunes-Ueno, everyone from the original ALLOW poetry group where some of the writing in this book was birthed, my parents, Mitch and Linda, and everyone whose kindness and care helped me cultivate resilience as a kid.

Big gratitude to you, the reader. I'm honored to be on this path of healing, and thriving, with you.

Finally, thank you to Adopt Me Rescue for choosing me to be Jake Billie Twist's forever human. Jake taught me about a kind of love I didn't even know existed, and he is the most perfect tiny scruffy service dog and best friend I could ever hope for.

NOTES

My Parents' Hell

1 Hymie Anisman, Amy Bombay, and Kim Matheson. "Intergenerational Trauma: Convergence of Multiple Processes among First Nations Peoples in Canada." *International Journal of Indigenous Health* 5, no. 3 (June 4, 2013). https://doi.org/https://jps.library .utoronto.ca/index.php/ijih/article/view/28987; Mallory E. Bowers and Rachel Yehuda. "Intergenerational Transmission of Stress in Humans." *Neuropsychopharmacology* 41, no. 1 (August 17, 2015): 232–44. https://doi.org/10.1038/npp.2015.247; Nader Perroud, Eugene Rutembesa, Ariane Paoloni-Giacobino, Jean Mutabaruka, Léon Mutesa, Ludwig Stenz, Alain Malafosse, and Félicien Karege. "The Tutsi Genocide and Transgenerational Transmission of Maternal Stress: Epigenetics and Biology of the HPA Axis." *World Journal of Biological Psychiatry* 15, no. 4 (April 2014): 334–45. https://doi.org/10.3109/15622975.2013.866693.

2 Rachel Yehuda and Amy Lehrner. "Intergenerational Transmission of Trauma Effects: Putative Role of Epigenetic Mechanisms." *World Psychiatry* 17, no. 3 (September 7, 2018): 243–57. https://doi.org/10.1002/wps.20568; Torsten Klengel, Brian G. Dias, and Kerry J. Ressler. "Models of Intergenerational and Transgenerational Transmission of Risk for Psychopathology in Mice."

Neuropsychopharmacology 41, no. 1 (August 18, 2015): 219–31. https://doi
.org/10.1038/npp.2015.249.

3   Kate M. Scott, Karestan C. Koenen, Sergio Aguilar-Gaxiola, Jordi
    Alonso, Matthias C. Angermeyer, Corina Benjet, Ronny Bruf-
    faerts, et al. "Associations between Lifetime Traumatic Events
    and Subsequent Chronic Physical Conditions: A Cross-National,
    Cross-Sectional Study." *PLoS ONE* 8, no. 11 (November 19, 2013).
    https://doi.org/10.1371/journal.pone.0080573; Steven E. Mock
    and Susan M. Arai. "Childhood Trauma and Chronic Illness in
    Adulthood: Mental Health and Socioeconomic Status as Explan-
    atory Factors and Buffers." *Frontiers in Psychology* 1 (January 31,
    2011). https://doi.org/10.3389/fpsyg.2010.00246; Robert F. Anda,
    David W. Brown, Shanta R. Dube, J. Douglas Bremner, Vincent J.
    Felitti, and Wayne H. Giles. "Adverse Childhood Experiences and
    Chronic Obstructive Pulmonary Disease in Adults." *American Jour-
    nal of Preventive Medicine* 34, no. 5 (May 2008): 396–403. https://doi
    .org/10.1016/j.amepre.2008.02.002.

4   Elmar W. Tobi, Roderick C. Slieker, René Luijk, Koen F. Dekkers,
    Aryeh D. Stein, Kate M. Xu, P. Eline Slagboom, Erik W. van Zwet, L.
    H. Lumey, and Bastiaan T. Heijmans. "DNA Methylation as a Medi-
    ator of the Association between Prenatal Adversity and Risk Factors
    for Metabolic Disease in Adulthood." *Science Advances* 4, no. 1 (Janu-
    ary 5, 2018). https://doi.org/10.1126/sciadv.aao4364.

5   P. Ekamper, F. van Poppel, A. D. Stein, and L. H. Lumey. "Indepen-
    dent and Additive Association of Prenatal Famine Exposure and
    Intermediary Life Conditions with Adult Mortality between Age
    18–63 Years." *Social Science & Medicine* 119 (October 2014): 232–39.
    https://doi.org/10.1016/j.socscimed.2013.10.027.

6   Linda M. Bierer, Heather N. Bader, Nikolaos P. Daskalakis,
    Amy Lehrner, Nadine Provençal, Tobias Wiechmann, Tor-
    sten Klengel, Iouri Makotkine, Elisabeth B. Binder, and Rachel
    Yehuda. "Intergenerational Effects of Maternal Holocaust

Exposure on Fkbp5 Methylation." *American Journal of Psychiatry* 177, no. 8 (August 1, 2020): 744–53. https://doi.org/10.1176/appi.ajp.2019.19060618.

7 Sophie Isobel, Melinda Goodyear, Trentham Furness, and Kim Foster. "Preventing Intergenerational Trauma Transmission: A Critical Interpretive Synthesis." *Journal of Clinical Nursing* 28, no. 7–8 (January 7, 2019): 1100–1113. https://doi.org/10.1111/jocn.14735.

Floating in the Swamp of Sadness

1 Meihua Yu, Lingling Huang, Jiaqi Mao, Gese DNA, and Siyang Luo. "Childhood Maltreatment, Automatic Negative Thoughts, and Resilience: The Protective Roles of Culture and Genes." *Journal of Interpersonal Violence* 37, no. 1–2 (March 19, 2020): 349–70. https://doi.org/10.1177/0886260520912582.

2 Saghar Chahar Mahali, Shadi Beshai, Justin R. Feeney, and Sandeep Mishra. "Associations of Negative Cognitions, Emotional Regulation, and Depression Symptoms across Four Continents: International Support for the Cognitive Model of Depression." *BMC Psychiatry* 20, no. 1 (January 13, 2020). https://doi.org/10.1186/s12888-019-2423-x.

Addiction: The Disease of Post-Trauma

1 Centers for Disease Control and Prevention. "Deaths from Excessive Alcohol Use in the United States," July 6, 2022. https://www.cdc.gov/alcohol/features/excessive-alcohol-deaths.html; NHTSA's National Center for Statistics and Analysis. "Alcohol-Impaired Driving." National Highway Traffic Safety Administration, April 2022. https://crashstats.nhtsa.dot.gov/Api/Public/ViewPublication/813294.

2 Centers for Disease Control and Prevention. "Heroin Overdose Data," June 6, 2022. https://www.cdc.gov/drugoverdose/deaths /heroin/index.html.

3 Kara R. Douglas, Grace Chan, Joel Gelernter, Albert J. Arias, Raymond F. Anton, Roger D. Weiss, Kathleen Brady, James Poling, Lindsay Farrer, and Henry R. Kranzler. "Adverse Childhood Events as Risk Factors for Substance Dependence: Partial Mediation by Mood and Anxiety Disorders." *Addictive Behaviors* 35, no. 1 (January 2010): 7–13. https://doi.org/10.1016 /j.addbeh.2009.07.004; Shanta R. Dube, Robert F. Anda, Vincent J. Felitti, Valerie J. Edwards, and Janet B. Croft. "Adverse Childhood Experiences and Personal Alcohol Abuse as an Adult." *Addictive Behaviors* 27, no. 5 (September 2002): 713–25. https://doi.org/10.1016 /s0306-4603(01)00204-0; Tara Strine. "Associations between Adverse Childhood Experiences, Psychological Distress, and Adult Alcohol Problems." *American Journal of Health Behavior* 36, no. 3 (2012). https://doi.org/10.5993/ajhb.36.3.11; Andreas Goebel, Emerson Krock, Clive Gentry, Mathilde R. Israel, Alexandra Jurczak, Carlos Morado Urbina, Katalin Sandor, et al. "Passive Transfer of Fibromyalgia Symptoms from Patients to Mice." *Journal of Clinical Investigation* 131, no. 13 (July 1, 2021). https://doi .org/10.1172/jci144201.

4 Catherine Stamoulis, Ross E. Vanderwert, Charles H. Zeanah, Nathan A. Fox, and Charles A. Nelson. "Early Psychosocial Neglect Adversely Impacts Developmental Trajectories of Brain Oscillations and Their Interactions." *Journal of Cognitive Neuroscience* 27, no. 12 (December 1, 2015): 2512–28. https://doi.org/10.1162 /jocn_a_00877; Center on the Developing Child. "InBrief: The Impact of Early Adversity on Child Development," 2007. https:// developingchild.harvard.edu/resources/inbrief-the-impact-of -early-adversity-on-childrens-development/; Julia I. Herzog and Christian Schmahl. "Adverse Childhood Experiences and the Consequences on Neurobiological, Psychosocial, and Somatic

Conditions across the Lifespan." *Frontiers in Psychiatry* 9 (September 4, 2018). https://doi.org/10.3389/fpsyt.2018.00420.

5 Office of the Associate Director for Communication. "Adverse Childhood Experiences (Aces)." Centers for Disease Control and Prevention. Accessed January 27, 2024. https://www.cdc.gov/vital signs/aces/index.html.

6 Héctor E. Alcalá, Ondine S. von Ehrenstein, and A. Janet Tomiyama. "Adverse Childhood Experiences and Use of Cigarettes and Smokeless Tobacco Products." *Journal of Community Health* 41, no. 5 (March 21, 2016): 969–76. https://doi.org/10.1007/s10900-016 -0179-5; Valerie J. Edwards, Robert F. Anda, David Gu, Shanta R. Dube, and Vincent J. Felitti. "Adverse Childhood Experiences and Smoking Persistence in Adults with Smoking-Related Symptoms and Illness." *Permanente Journal* 11, no. 2 (June 2007): 5–13. https:// doi.org/10.7812/tpp/06-110.

7 Rosalie Broekhof, Hans M. Nordahl, Lars Tanum, and Sara G. Selvik. "Adverse Childhood Experiences and Their Association with Substance Use Disorders in Adulthood: A General Population Study (Young-Hunt)." *Addictive Behaviors Reports* 17 (June 2023): 100488. https://doi.org/10.1016/j.abrep.2023.100488.

8 Robert F. Anda, David W. Brown, Shanta R. Dube, J. Douglas Bremner, Vincent J. Felitti, and Wayne H. Giles. "Adverse Childhood Experiences and Chronic Obstructive Pulmonary Disease in Adults." *American Journal of Preventive Medicine* 34, no. 5 (May 2008): 396–403. https://doi.org/10.1016/j.amepre.2008.02.002.

9 Karen Hughes, Mark A. Bellis, Katherine A. Hardcastle, Dinesh Sethi, Alexander Butchart, Christopher Mikton, Lisa Jones, and Michael P. Dunne. "The Effect of Multiple Adverse Childhood Experiences on Health: A Systematic Review and Meta-Analysis." *Lancet Public Health* 2, no. 8 (August 2017). https://doi.org/10.1016 /s2468-2667(17)30118-4.

10 David W. Brown, Robert F. Anda, Henning Tiemeier, Vincent J. Felitti, Valerie J. Edwards, Janet B. Croft, and Wayne H. Giles.

"Adverse Childhood Experiences and the Risk of Premature Mortality." *American Journal of Preventive Medicine* 37, no. 5 (November 2009): 389–96. https://doi.org/10.1016/j.amepre.2009.06.021.

11 Phillip W. Schnarrs, Amy L. Stone, Robert Salcido, Aleta Baldwin, Charlotte Georgiou, and Charles B. Nemeroff. "Differences in Adverse Childhood Experiences (ACEs) and Quality of Physical and Mental Health between Transgender and Cisgender Sexual Minorities." *Journal of Psychiatric Research* 119 (December 2019): 1–6. https://doi.org/10.1016/j.jpsychires.2019.09.001; Judith P. Andersen and John Blosnich. "Disparities in Adverse Childhood Experiences among Sexual Minority and Heterosexual Adults: Results from a Multi-State Probability-Based Sample." *PLoS ONE* 8, no. 1 (January 23, 2013). https://doi.org/10.1371/journal.pone.0054691; Melissa S. Jones, Hayley Pierce, and Kevin Shafer. "Gender Differences in Early Adverse Childhood Experiences and Youth Psychological Distress." *Journal of Criminal Justice* 83 (November 2022): 101925. https://doi.org/10.1016/j.jcrimjus.2022.101925; Office of the Associate Director for Communication. "Adverse Childhood Experiences (ACEs)." Centers for Disease Control and Prevention. Accessed January 27, 2024. https://www.cdc.gov/vitalsigns/aces/index.html.

12 Patrick Olivieri, Bruce Solitar, and Michel Dubois. "Childhood Risk Factors for Developing Fibromyalgia." *Open Access Rheumatology: Research and Reviews*, December 2012, 109. https://doi.org/10.2147/oarrr.s36086; Lucas C. Godoy, Claudia Frankfurter, Matthew Cooper, Christine Lay, Robert Maunder, and Michael E. Farkouh. "Association of Adverse Childhood Experiences with Cardiovascular Disease Later in Life." *JAMA Cardiology* 6, no. 2 (February 1, 2021): 228. https://doi.org/10.1001/jamacardio.2020.6050; Shanta R. Dube, DeLisa Fairweather, William S. Pearson, Vincent J. Felitti, Robert F. Anda, and Janet B. Croft. "Cumulative Childhood Stress and Autoimmune Diseases in Adults." *Psychosomatic*

Medicine 71, no. 2 (February 2009): 243–50. https://doi.org/10.1097/psy.obo13e3181907888;   E. Von Cheong, Carol Sinnott, Darren Dahly, and Patricia M. Kearney. "Adverse Childhood Experiences (ACES) and Later-Life Depression: Perceived Social Support as a Potential Protective Factor." *BMJ Open* 7, no. 9 (September 2017). https://doi.org/10.1136/bmjopen-2016-013228; Christina M. van der Feltz-Cornelis, Evelien C. Potters, Anniek van Dam, Rachel P. M. Koorndijk, Iman Elfeddali, and Jonna F. van Eck van der Sluijs. "Adverse Childhood Experiences (ACE) in Outpatients with Anxiety and Depressive Disorders and Their Association with Psychiatric and Somatic Comorbidity and Revictimization. Cross-Sectional Observational Study." *Journal of Affective Disorders* 246 (March 2019): 458–64. https://doi.org/10.1016/j.jad.2018.12.096; Hui Liao, Chaoyang Yan, Ying Ma, and Jing Wang. "Impact of Adverse Childhood Experiences on Older Adult Poverty: Mediating Role of Depression." *Frontiers in Public Health* 9 (November 5, 2021). https://doi.org/10.3389/fpubh.2021.749640.

13 Vincent J. Felitti, Robert F. Anda, Dale Nordenberg, David F. Williamson, Alison M. Spitz, Valerie Edwards, Mary P. Koss, and James S. Marks. "Relationship of Childhood Abuse and Household Dysfunction to Many of the Leading Causes of Death in Adults." *American Journal of Preventive Medicine* 14, no. 4 (May 1998): 245–58. https://doi.org/10.1016/s0749-3797(98)00017-8.

14 Chantel L. Daines, Dustin Hansen, M. Lelinneth Novilla, and AliceAnn Crandall. "Effects of Positive and Negative Childhood Experiences on Adult Family Health." *BMC Public Health* 21, no. 1 (April 5, 2021). https://doi.org/10.1186/s12889-021-10732-w.

15 Mark A. Bellis, Katie Hardcastle, Kat Ford, Karen Hughes, Kathryn Ashton, Zara Quigg, and Nadia Butler. "Does Continuous Trusted Adult Support in Childhood Impart Life-Course Resilience against Adverse Childhood Experiences: A Retrospective Study on Adult Health-Harming Behaviours and Mental

Well-Being." *BMC Psychiatry* 17, no. 1 (March 23, 2017). https://doi
.org/10.1186/s12888-017-1260-z.

16 Robert C. Whitaker, Tracy Dearth-Wesley, and Allison N. Herman.
"Childhood Family Connection and Adult Flourishing: Associations across Levels of Childhood Adversity." *Academic Pedi-
atrics* 21, no. 8 (November 2021): 1380–87. https://doi.org/10.1016
/j.acap.2021.03.002.

17 Egon Bachler, Alexander Frühmann, Herbert Bachler, Benjamin
Aas, Marius Nickel, and Guenter Karl Schiepek. "The Effect of
Childhood Adversities and Protective Factors on the Development of Child-Psychiatric Disorders and Their Treatment." *Frontiers in Psychology* 9 (November 15, 2018). https://doi.org/10.3389
/fpsyg.2018.02226.

18 Rachel Yehuda, Nikolaos P. Daskalakis, Linda M. Bierer, Heather
N. Bader, Torsten Klengel, Florian Holsboer, and Elisabeth B.
Binder. "Holocaust Exposure Induced Intergenerational Effects
on FKBP5 Methylation." *Biological Psychiatry* 80, no. 5 (September
2016): 372–80. https://doi.org/10.1016/j.biopsych.2015.08.005.

19 Dora L. Costa, Noelle Yetter, and Heather DeSomer. "Intergen-
erational Transmission of Paternal Trauma among US Civil War
Ex-POWs." *Proceedings of the National Academy of Sciences* 115, no. 44
(October 15, 2018): 11215–20. https://doi.org/10.1073/pnas.1803630115.

20 Steven J. Micheletti, Kasia Bryc, Samantha G. Ancona Esselmann,
William A. Freyman, Meghan E. Moreno, G. David Poznik, Anjali
J. Shastri, et al. "Genetic Consequences of the Transatlantic Slave
Trade in the Americas." *American Journal of Human Genetics* 107, no.
2 (August 2020): 265–77. https://doi.org/10.1016/j.ajhg.2020.06.012.

The Migraine Years

1 Robert Anda, Gretchen Tietjen, Elliott Schulman, Vincent
Felitti, and Janet Croft. "Adverse Childhood Experiences and

Frequent Headaches in Adults." *Headache: The Journal of Head and Face Pain* 50, no. 9 (October 2010): 1473–81. https://doi.org /10.1111/j.1526-4610.2010.01756.x.

Spoons

1 Christine Miserandino. "The Spoon Theory Written by Christine Miserandino." But You Don't Look Sick, April 26, 2013. https:// butyoudontlooksick.com/articles/written-by-christine/the-spoon -theory/.

My Fucking Back Hurts

1 Mohamed Jarraya, Ali Guermazi, Amanda L. Lorbergs, Elana Brochin, Douglas P. Kiel, Mary L. Bouxsein, L. Adrienne Cupples, and Elizabeth J. Samelson. "A Longitudinal Study of Disc Height Narrowing and Facet Joint Osteoarthritis at the Thoracic and Lumbar Spine, Evaluated by Computed Tomography: The Framingham Study." *Spine Journal* 18, no. 11 (November 2018): 2065–73. https://doi.org/10.1016/j.spinee.2018.04.010.

2 *Pain Brain*. Accessed June 14, 2023. https://painbrainfilm.com.

3 Benjamin Mosch, Verena Hagena, Stephan Herpertz, Michaela Ruttorf, and Martin Diers. "Neural Correlates of Control over Pain in Fibromyalgia Patients." *NeuroImage: Clinical* 37 (February 19, 2023): 103355. https://doi.org/10.1016/j.nicl.2023.103355.

4 Mosch et al. "Neural Correlates of Control over Pain."

5 Amir Minerbi, Emmanuel Gonzalez, Nicholas Brereton, Mary-Ann Fitzcharles, Stéphanie Chevalier, and Yoram Shir. "Altered Serum Bile Acid Profile in Fibromyalgia Is Associated with Specific Gut Microbiome Changes and Symptom Severity." *Pain* 164, no. 2 (May 19, 2022). https://doi.org/10.1097/j.pain.0000000000002694; Amir Minerbi, Emmanuel Gonzalez, Nicholas J. B. Brereton, Abraham

Anjarkouchian, Ken Dewar, Mary-Ann Fitzcharles, Stéphanie Chevalier, and Yoram Shir. "Altered Microbiome Composition in Individuals with Fibromyalgia." *Pain* 160, no. 11 (June 18, 2019): 2589–2602. https://doi.org/10.1097/j.pain.0000000000001640.

6 Sharon Reynolds. "Retraining the Brain to Treat Chronic Pain." National Institutes of Health, November 9, 2021. https://www.nih.gov/news-events/nih-research-matters/retraining-brain-treat-chronic-pain.

A Mother's Love

1 Rachael Maddox. "Chapter 1." In *ReBloom: Archetypal Trauma Resolution for Personal & Collective Healing*, 32–32. Rachael Maddox, LLC, 2021.

Hacking Human Suffering

1 David Halberstam and Daniel Joseph Singal. *The Making of a Quagmire: America and Vietnam during the Kennedy Era.* Lanham, MD: Rowman & Littlefield, 2008, 288.

2 Devon Price, PhD. *Laziness Does Not Exist.* New York: Atria Books, 2020.

Gold Linings

1 Cristina A. Fernandez, Karmel W. Choi, Brandon D. L. Marshall, Benjamin Vicente, Sandra Saldivia, Robert Kohn, Karestan C. Koenen, Kristopher L. Arheart, and Stephen L. Buka. "Assessing the Relationship between Psychosocial Stressors and Psychiatric Resilience among Chilean Disaster Survivors." *British Journal of Psychiatry* 217, no. 5 (2020): 630–37. https://doi.org/10.1192/bjp.2020.88.

2 Kathryn M. Magruder, Katie A. McLaughlin, and Diane L. Elmore Borbon. "Trauma Is a Public Health Issue." *European Journal of Psychotraumatology* 8, no. 1 (January 1, 2017). https://doi.org/10.1080 /20008198.2017.1375338.

3 Andrew Carlins. "From Silver to Gold Lining; from Comparative to True Gratitude." Kenan Institute for Ethics at Duke University, October 31, 2019. https://kenan.ethics.duke.edu/from-silver -to-gold-lining-from-comparative-to-true-gratitude.

4 Richard G. Tedeschi and Lawrence G. Calhoun. "The Post-traumatic Growth Inventory: Measuring the Positive Legacy of Trauma." *Journal of Traumatic Stress* 9, no. 3 (July 1996): 455–71. https://doi.org/10.1007/bf02103658.

5 Richard G. Tedeschi, and Lawrence G. Calhoun. "The Post-traumatic Growth Inventory: Measuring the Positive Legacy of Trauma." *Journal of Traumatic Stress* 9, no. 3 (January 1996): 455–71. https://doi.org/10.1002/jts.2490090305.

6 Albert Camus. *Personal Writings.* New York: Vintage Books, 2020, 320.

INDEX

ABOUT THE AUTHOR

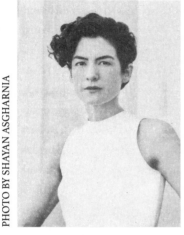

Jessica Graham is a certified somatic trauma-resolution guide and trained Brainspotting practitioner, specializing in complex-PTSD and post-traumatic growth. Jessica is also a meditation teacher, sex, relationship, and spiritual guide for couples and individuals, chronic pain coach, a senior teacher in Shinzen Young's mindfulness system, and the author of *Good Sex: Getting Off without Checking Out*. They have offered workshops at various centers internationally, including Esalen Institute, and their work can also be found on many apps and in The Great Courses' Masters of Mindfulness. In addition to this, Jessica is an award-winning actor and filmmaker. They live between Los Angeles and Philadelphia, with the world's best tiny scruffy dog. *Being (Sick) Enough* is their second book. Connect with Jessica, known as "Jess," at jessica graham.com.

ABOUT NORTH ATLANTIC BOOKS

North Atlantic Books (NAB) is an independent, nonprofit publisher committed to a bold exploration of the relationships between mind, body, spirit, and nature. Founded in 1974, NAB aims to nurture a holistic view of the arts, sciences, humanities, and healing. To make a donation or to learn more about our books, authors, events, and newsletter, please visit www.northatlanticbooks.com.